Memoirs of Madness

Christopher Markowski

ISBN: 1491027819
ISBN-13: 978-1491027813

ACKNOWLEDGMENTS

To my parents, who endured and still cared for me through my hellish journey. To my lovely wife Megan, who was there to bring me out of the depths of hell

Prologue

I have had my engagement with the abyss and the monsters
of this world. Growing up I often ran into encounters in which I
was seen as inferior by people. I was a good kid, but the world
would have none of that when it came to me. I was the shy type,
maybe too timid. I sat and listened when others babbled on with
their version of how it is, what is good, what is not. I wasn't
outspoken, as such nobody ever knew what I thought. It didn't
matter to them though, after all, I was just a child. My
classmates were more opinionated that me. Eventually as I
gained pubescence, I began to feel the pressures of the outside
world crash down upon my head and I had enough of it. Enter,
my rebellious era. But something more kicked in before that was
ever settled, something that has deeply affected the core of my
self forever. It has interrupted my path and sent me upon a new
one. Today I write these words a new man, on this same path.
Having hopefully conquered or at least quelled a searing madness

that ripped through my bone and flesh at a very critical time in any young man's life, the early 20's. All of this has made me a better person and due to this I am a subscriber to the old saying "what doesn't kill you, makes you stronger". I have come away from this story wondering how I didn't get myself killed or kill someone during this phenomenal fervor, an out of control imagination. An imagination that ran amok overcame me and I created a world as entirely different as it could possibly be, yet still somehow managed to walk around this planet and interacting with daily life not realizing I was living out my own dark subconscious fantasy, or perhaps, nightmare at times. I have learned many lessons from this and hope those families who may experience this in loved ones, as it is all too common a theme, can find insight into what their own are experiencing and possibly be able to cope themselves. For those experiencing it now, I find no reason they would stumble on this book, unless it may be during a brief moment of clarity; but those who experienced what I have, do not of course have reason to peruse this first-hand account of mental illness, because they would be have already experienced a similar state of mind. That is if they are cognizant enough to remember, which luckily I am. In writing this I have confronted my manic thoughts head on instead of burying them in some dark recess of my mind that may only wreak havoc later. I would ask that those who experience the similar states of mind that I bring before you in these memoirs, that you too confront your past demons as well, in whatever way you are apt to. Contemplation and writing have brought me to conquer the maniacal memories that could very much have rooted me in a lasting insecurity of social instability and awkwardness.

The difference between truly believing and knowing isn't much different to many. When this occurs with mental illness, there is no difference. When I was God there was nothing better; no better feeling before it nothing will ever compare to the glory of myself that I had in my own mind. My sense of superiority was to the *nth* degree and could go no further. My emotions were euphoric and blissful, nothing we can do on this planet, no goals can be met (becoming the world leader, becoming the wealthiest person in the world, or anything similar to that), could compare to what I was experiencing. We do this reality trick with kids a bit with Santa Clause, he doesn't exist, but they believe he does, and it's very, very fun for kids. If only the experience of feeling all powerful, as I did while my mania was at its peak, could be sustained indefinitely; I would still like to experience this feeling I had without any ill effect. If it could be sustained through the rest of my life, actually believing I was God and even hallucinating the effects of my own that I created, which I did. If I was single and had nobody to care for who know me as the sane individual I do now, I might be willing to make that trade of total disillusionment for reality. Would I be happier? Possibly, I might even be in ecstasy. But there are also the deep, utterly abysmal periods of despair and hopelessness that I experienced. Knowing what I know now, I would never choose to go back. I couldn't. Since my episode, which lasted a few years in its peak stages, I have pursued real world knowledge in the form of logic, science, and philosophy. My goal to seek truth and knowledge in all areas was a means to overcome the disillusioned reality I had already lived out. I was sick and tired of fantasy as I had lived it and I knew I had to get my head on straight. Would that be the sole result of my reaction to my illness, or was it what I was to scratch an itch of intellectual curiosity, regardless of my plight? Of course I would never know that, but it doesn't matter now anyways. The experience has changed me for the better and the old adage *"what doesn't kill you, makes you stronger"* applies perfectly for me and this instance. Now hopefully I can help by providing my story to the world and possibly just as important, hopefully I can also eliminate some stigma.

Chapter 1

Sitting outside on my back porch I watched the grass slowly wave in the gentle breeze. It was a typical hot, sunny day. The motion of the grass was particularly hypnotizing for some reason. The wind caressed the blades in a rhythmic wave that provided an image of a flowing sea of green. This rhythm of nature seemed to be some sort of communication possibly. I needed to find something to help me figure out my current situation, which was inexplicably doomed. I was certainly in a precarious situation, one in which I was absolutely positive I would be spending all of eternity in eternal damnation and fire. How I got here I wasn't too sure, but I was sure that it seemed to be my destiny. I heard the demons roaring outside now, they have possessed my neighbors. It's a shame because they were quite amicable. It seems the entire world is going to hell, as other random people outside start growling demonically that walk by my houses sidewalk. Someone passes by in their car and I heard a demon that sounded as if it were born of fire, utter out a guttural yell that should make everyone in the neighborhood begin packing their bags. For me, however, I was in a rather catatonic state of mind listening to all of this. I figured they may terrify the remaining un-possessed souls of the neighborhood, but I already knew I was doomed and had a clue to decipher. I reaffixed my attention on the rhythm of the grass and listened intently at the wind for their instructions. Nature was seemingly quite knowledgeable on my predicament. The rhythmic sign language of the grass and the whispers of the wind were always very agreeable to me. Yet they seem to only be agreeing with me because nature itself is afraid of me.

Meanwhile these demonic outburst coming from the neighborhood was rather unsettling and yet very interesting, as long as they left me alone and only taunted me verbally that is. I was completely calm hearing these loud, disturbing voices from my poor neighbors. I guess they weren't so good after all I thought. I had already been through quite the ride of hell at this point, so dealing with demonic possessions of half the town wasn't very worrisome considering what I've been through. One thing is for certain, I need to get use to hell. I took my socks off and let them roast on the sidewalk that was heated by that inferno of a sun. If only I could start getting used to the inevitable hellfire awaiting me, maybe it would make it easier. I then thought, it's probably useless, God would probably turn up the heat as soon as I got comfortable anyways, exponentially. Such is life. I went back inside my parent's house, where I could then commence my communication with the outside world through telepathy and television, because I was the antichrist and had some pretty nice powers. I guess that's the perk of being guaranteed the darkest fate of all time.

Chapter 2

I was always a little different. As a young kid in grade school I sensed I was a little off, but that was ok. I once had my parents question my teachers about my questionable drawings, which were of monsters. After that meeting I thought something may be wrong with me. I was quiet, but one thing my mother saw of me that was peculiar was that I didn't ask questions. I just did what I was told, listened and accepted everything as how they were presented to me. Of course, I didn't know better. Other kids would be running around, talking, asking. But I was rather subdued and introverted from a very young age. I don't know why exactly that was the case for me, but perhaps it was because I thought I didn't know better. I *knew* that I didn't know anything. I had a few odd feelings growing up that I remember vividly.

One evening I got out of bed, I had to be about 4 or 5 and saw my parents in the living room. Dad was watching TV, Mom reading a book, things were exactly as they should have been. However everything was very odd, disturbing almost. I felt something very peculiar. It was more than just being ill or with a fever, as if everything was very scary. To me, my parents even seemed scary. The house was terribly scary as well, the furniture, and particularly the frog vase in the living room holding some plant that smelled like fresh soil. Why I was paranoid of everything, I did not know. My perception had changed for apparently no reason whatsoever. I encountered a much more intense feeling like this years later, which may very well be defined now as a panic attack. Another instance was a terrible dream I had. It wasn't quite a nightmare as it wasn't very terrifying, but it was rather disturbing to me. I had to have been about the same age, maybe a little older. I was in bed asleep; however there was another me in bed. He was laying just the opposite of me with his feet to mine laying down, his head towards the foot of the bed. Not only was he another me, he was my opposite and he was evil. I remember in the dream being paralyzed in my bed, with him right there, thinking of what to do. It was my anti-me, a little terrifying version of myself sleeping in my bed. I quickly rose up and he did the same and we began choking each other. *One of us had to die.* I don't remember how it ended, but in retrospect, it could be seen as who I had inside of me. That being a scary, delusional, evil being that would come out of me, to be completely out of control and insane. This person would not think rationally at all. He would be completely paranoid and delusional. He would be reckless and careless of everything and everyone around him and would be very dangerous to all, including himself. Before this person came out and took over the *real* me, I would read and hear about bad guys, criminals, murderers, all the bizarre things people do that could be described as sheer evil and wonder just what kind of mindset they would have. Little did I know of course that I would experience that type of mindset first hand, and I would have to fight that evil person that rest inside of me, who so interrupted my sleep one night.

My parents were much older than I was, this being one of that factors I learned later that increased the likelihood of mental illness. My father was born right in the middle of the Great Depression, 1925, in the city of Chicago. He told me stories of how his father would have to try to eke out a living by selling newspapers. I, being born in 1979, thought that must've been terrible. I grew up in an era when 13 year olds were the ones who delivered papers, while riding their bikes through the neighborhood before school. He later moved to the farm in Shelby, Indiana and became a country boy, taking up hunting and fishing. He passed those experiences on to me. I learned a lot of good from my father, but there was a downside. He had a terrible temper and was overbearing as I was growing up and trying to gain my own identity. I hated him for a period of time even though the reason he protected me from the outside world so much was because he loved me. He wanted me to stay out of trouble, but he tried to hard to do so. At his age, he was very out of tune with the modern world in my viewpoint. My friends were all being raised with younger parents and were more lax with their rules, which made my perspective of my father to be that much stricter. Disobedience was intolerable and was met with a whipping with a belt. When I was older, sometimes it was with the buckle on the end. It was his old fashioned way of parenting in an era where that type of treatment of your children was beginning to become frowned upon. The age of my father and his overbearing nature seem to be to key aspects that elevated my risk for mental illness when I was to reach my early 20's.

My mother on the other hand, being a little younger than my father, was born in 1938. She had her own contribution to my risk factor. Of course I don't blame my parents for what happened to me, some things in life just happen and we have to work through them. Growing up with two older parents, people who didn't know me thought they were my grandparents. What I know of my mother's contribution to my risk factor is genetic, in that when I was a young boy, possibly in first or second grade, my mother having a nervous breakdown after the death of my father's son from a previous marriage. He was murdered in Chicago and it was a too grisly for my mother to come to terms with. I was only 5 years old when I found out, which came from a phone call that my dad received one wintry night. My dad was furious and broken, but apparently when my mother learned of the details she couldn't handle it. She was too sensitive at the time, something that must have changed afterwards, because I remember being rather hardened in her old age. Shortly after my half brothers death, I remember my mom having issues of being paranoid of werewolves and other monsters. My father talked to me about it a little bit, but of course I wasn't given that much information. My mother ended up having an extended hospital stay for a few weeks. During that time it was just my father and I at home, which was very odd to me. I didn't know exactly what was going on but my dad was able to comfort me enough to know everything would be alright, which he ended up being correct. I never really knew of another mental breakdown that my mother had and she was relatively a normal mom throughout the rest of her life. Obviously to me, her genetic make up made her prone to this sort mental breakdown as it seems to have been passed on to myself. Coupled with my father being as old as he is and I being the youngest, perhaps that is why it explains how I would one day find myself in a complete psychotic breakdown.

Once I had graduated high school, I had had enough of my parents. I had taken up drinking with some friends and found what was missing from the rest of my life, the other side of a "good", disciplined Catholic upbringing. I was no exploring everything I had never been allowed to previously. This included heavy metal music, drinking, and a little marijuana here and there. Curious in this other world I had been introduced to, I was eager to try anything at least once. I was a typical "bad" teenager at that point; I had already ditched quite a few days of class at my Catholic High school and had gotten caught. My grades had dropped considerably each year of high school as well as I began to reject authority of all type, which had a direct correlation to my over authoritative father. As I began my descent into the darkest vices of life, my father and I had already been in a few physical confrontations as a result of both of our stubbornness. However, I was no longer suspect to any physical lashings from a belt as I was now nearing full physical development and my father was in his 70's. He was no longer able to control me physically. His temper however persisted and even seemed to increase as he got older. It seemed his mental health was deteriorating as well, which my mother too had her issues with his temper and controlling nature. He had problems remembering things, was getting to be repetitive and was often crude and rather crass, saying anything that came to his mind. I would garner that he was also experiencing some delirium as well, his old mind was failing him and it may have always had its issues to begin with. I understand his mother, my grandmother, whom I only remember seeing on her death bed, was quite the mean old lady. Apparently my father inherited that from her as well. There was some suspicion that my father might have been bipolar, but he was old enough to get away with acting however he wanted, especially in public. This may be the reason why it went undiagnosed. I did realize later though that my mother ended up getting him some anti psychotic medicines later in his life after I had moved out.

Chapter 3

I remember my mental illness beginning when I lost my first job that could be considered a career. I'm sure I had problems before this, but none this discernable. I was the Golden Boy of this company, excelling on their largest account and doing the work of at least 2 people. I was well respected by my 8th month with the company, and I was only 20 years old. I was making good money and working quite a bit of overtime, laboring at a desk job for 60-70 hours per week. Then on my 13th month I got fired, for no good reason that I could conceive. It was possibly because I was raking in too much overtime. The shock of being fired after putting in so much effort and accomplishing so much in just a little period of time really took its toll on me. I was shattered and didn't know what to do next, except try to find something else. Hopefully the little experience that I garnered could propel me elsewhere, but the outlook was grim for me, without a college degree and having to start all over at some job that might pay just over minimum wage. I cried when I was fired because my foolish 20 year old self had thought I had just embarked on a career that would propel me to greatness in the business world one day. I was too young to understand life is full of challenges of this manner and became too confident too fast. This contributed to the stress I endured after being terminated. Coupled with still trying to find my own identify as a man, I was now faced with the realization that I would have to now stay at home with my parents being jobless and soon to be out of money.

Back at home I was still attempting to move out on my own and get another job as quickly as possible. I looked for months, online, in the newspapers but had no luck. Having the high expectations I set for myself and failing miserably, I was gradually reduced to walking around my home in a daze, not talking to my parents, smoking a lot of pot and playing the card game "spades" online. I was living a directionless life as I had given up hope. The lack of finding work and my sadness from being a bum propelled me into an unexpected depression, which I have never experienced before. I didn't see it coming as a result and didn't realize what was even happening to me. I know I ended up walking around the house in a daze, aimlessly doing nothing. I looked like I just got hit by a train after 5 months of joblessness. After some time of this, I ended up getting an email back from one of my old co workers. He talked me into reapplying at the company for a different position in the warehouse. One of the managers in the warehouse who I always worked well with wanted to hire me back. He too thought I was unjustly fired and knew I was a good worker, so I got a job at my old company. I started on for less pay of course, but was happy to be working again and had hope that I could climb up the ladder fairly easily again. For whatever reason, this is when the mania kicked in. Perhaps it was due to being happy a bit too fast after a harsh depression as well as a genetic predisposition, but when it kicked in, it was as if I was no longer the same person, but someone completely different. This all happened very rapidly and the symptoms were very severe, to which none of those who knew me closest were given any warning signs. That probably has something to do with my introverted nature, but nonetheless this is a very scary aspect of what happened to me and part of the reason why it was so dangerous.

Shortly after starting the new job, I remember crazy thoughts occurring during my second stint at work.   I was around the age of 22 and trying to learn a new position that I really had no experience or knowledge of whatsoever. People that were below me in rank at status were suddenly telling me what to do and how to do it.   On my way to work each day I would listen to music and suddenly began to think that all the lyrics were meant for me. I could hear voices and they were coming from people I knew and people I didn't know. I thought I had extra sensory perception (ESP) and was hearing their thoughts. I worked a couple days there. During work I would hear some voices over the PA system and they were about me. They were thanking me for coming back, and how I was now here to save the company. I was thankful that they were so happy to have me back. Little did I know this was all just my hallucination and it was a hallucination that made me manic and grandiose. I bought into it hook line and sinker, never thinking that what I wasn't sensing couldn't possibly be reality. After my first week of work, I was looking forward to the weekend and celebrating my new found glory at my job, as well as this intriguing psychic ability I was developing. The depression to the mania was a little too much for me to handle, but I didn't know that at the time. I was hearing voices everywhere; it was intense that Saturday morning. I was driving aimlessly listening to my music loud, focusing on these telepathic powers flowing through my mind. There were so many at a time that I couldn't understand it what everyone was saying. I needed to find a way to control this, so I continued trying to focus on making out what exactly all these voices were saying. I would go on drives to nowhere just so I could smoke pot, listen to music, and use my ESP. I realized the marijuana made the voices come through more clearly, to the point where I can actually make sense of it. I'd drive all day that Saturday, driving hours to another state, not realizing where I was going but not caring. Suddenly someone in the highway across the divider gave me an angry telepathic message. *Who are you to talk like that to me?* Not sure just what driver it was, I rolled down my window, stuck my hand out and flipped off everyone I saw, for miles.

Chapter 4

Due to the rapid progression of hearing voices and the amount of voices, the way I processed this in my reality is that people were communicating to me with their thoughts now and had no need to speak. Not only did I have ESP, everyone did, and it was all because of me. I was the link that gave everybody the ability to read each others minds. There was no rhyme or reason as to why I thought these things; it was just what came to my mind. This reasoning wasn't inductive to calming me down. My belief in my own rationality was solid, to the point where it wasn't a belief anymore, but fact. I was ramping up to a point where something would end up giving. I didn't know it, but these type of thought processes cannot sustain without having something either very severe occur, to myself or others. By the time I got tired of flipping everyone off while driving for miles, I was also tired of driving. I headed home, exhausted mentally and physically from my telepathic usage. *My bed awaits and a new promising day tomorrow.*

Sunday came quickly; I didn't sleep much being in this manic state. I learned of a Carnival being held after visiting a friend in the morning for another bag of marijuana and some video games. After learning of this carnival, I thought that it was being held in my honor, after all, I had recently given everyone the power to communicate telepathically, and this delighted me immensely. I went by myself as my friends invited me to meet them there. Once there things went wrong. There were too many people there, too much noise and my senses weren't capable of handling the stress of being at the carnival. For some reason I didn't like this carnival that was in my honor. I perceived the people around me, who neglected to acknowledge the power I had given them, as being very pretentious. Perhaps they were trying to trick me or surprise me later, keeping it calm in order to develop a plot against me. I then started to *act* like I was special because I felt neglected that I wasn't getting the attention I deserved. *After all, you people all have ESP because of me, damn it.* I was hitting on all the women there, which is completely not my normal nature. I ended up becoming completely nervous due to this fact that nobody seemed to care that I gave them ESP. I felt like, since they had this power, they no longer needed me. Now this is all interesting, because I was able to reason correctly about my unreasonable thoughts, so why couldn't I process that my blatantly unreasonable thoughts were irrational?

On my way home voices entered my head that everything was free for me since I gave humanity the power of telepathy. They didn't want to talk to me there because my gift for giving everyone this power would be that they would communicate to me (as they were now) that I would never have to pay for everything again. Low on gas and happy about this gift communicated to me by the voices I drove into the gas station. I nodded at the clerk as to say hi, I'm here for the free gas as promised. He nodded back. I filled up and slowly pulled out into the street at the corner red light, waiting for green. The next thing I know this guy comes out of nowhere and slaps me in the face through my open window of my truck. Well, things went from bliss to ferocious anger in split seconds. I got out of my truck and proceeded to punch this man repeatedly, without ever looking at who he was. All I know is that he slapped me, in the middle of the street with cars all around us. The man quickly gave up, putting his hands in the air and told me to calm down, which I did. I was a merciful telepathic being. Having found power in my new found ability, I waited calmly for the police to come because after all, this guy slapped me for no reason. Besides, I needed to talk to the authorities as we should probably work together on my upcoming world takeover. They arrived and I calmly took a seat in the passenger seat of the squad car. I talked to the officer, but of course mentally. It seemed he wasn't understanding my mind so I continued to tell him how my amazing powers of giving ESP was so big that we needed to contact the media, the chief of police, the mayor, the president, whomever. Then suddenly my parents drove up to the intersection. Did the police call them or was this purely by chance? *Oh right, they are aware telepathically as I probably transmitted out subconsciously what was going on to everyone.* It's odd little coincidences like this that made me believe in my own delusions even further. I never did find out the answer to this question as to how they showed just as I was having a breakdown in the middle of that intersection. I imagine it was by coincidence as it was along a well- travelled road. My parents were backed away by the officer and I sort of shrugged my head, believing they were hearing my thoughts and would understand that everything is going to be ok. *Hell, everything is going to be great, I am famous!* Soon after my parents arrived, an ambulance showed up. I initially thought it was for the person I had punched, I hoped he didn't have any internal damage. The officer got out and opened my side of the door and escorted me to the ambulance. I glanced over at my parents were out of the car, and they looked so sad and confused, but I didn't know why. I waved goodbye and stepped into the ambulance, and asked for a cup of water. They said they didn't have any. *Well that's just the most ridiculous thing I heard all day.* I proceeded to complain to the paramedics about why these damn ambulances don't come prepared with water for people to drink and how it's a life necessity. They just stared at me rather bewildered. I never questioned at the moment why I was going in an ambulance, for some unknown reason it didn't cross my mind at the time.

Chapter 5

Upon arriving at the hospital, a new animal came over me. For some reason, I don't know why, I began to believe I was the gatekeeper to the keys of Heaven and hell and that when I died the world ended for everyone. The only chance for women to get into Heaven is if they had sex with me and the only chance for men to get into hell is if they had sex with me. I then sent out an ESP message to all men that I wasn't going to have sex with any men so you're all going to hell. I kind of laughed at that... A terrifying image of the bowels of hell came to my mind. It was terribly frightening and was even more afraid I was going there. The nurse asked me some questions and answered them the best I could, but I was utterly confused at all these things racing across my mind. I have no idea what was asked or what was said, and eventually I was led to my room by a nurse. I was thinking she was trying to gain entrance into heaven, that she too knew what was going on. Somehow that didn't happen and I went to my room alone. *Well maybe she just hadn't had enough persuasion yet, after all this new found power of mine is new to everyone.*

It was a calm evening, serene and peaceful at the mental ward of St. Margaret's Hospital. I was in my bed lying down, looking at the wooden door, just staring at it in a spaced out mood. Suddenly the wood began to move and an image formed.

It became the image of some perverted cartoon man who camouflaged perfectly into the wood door. *Surely I was the only one who could see this. It must be some sort of message for me.* As it turned out though, this little wooden man was here to bother me, to pester me, and was likely sent by some demons just to annoy me. Why, I didn't know. I closed my eyes but opened them again and there he was *masturbating* in the door and laughing at me. *Why was he doing this?* It was funny at all. I looked away to try to make it go away again, but there he was persisting. His wood grain body and his devilish grin while he did his little dirty deed troubled me. Then, I noticed how terrible I smelled... I needed a shower. This got my mind off the door and I turned over and tried to go to sleep. My mind raced with thoughts that I couldn't control, from all angles. More telepathic communications occurred with world leaders, famous people, and the people still hanging out in the hallway of the hospital annex that I stayed. Who knows how long I stayed up doing this, but sleep wasn't what I was interested in. I was interested in achieving the power I was guaranteed through my divine nature and incredible telepathic mind.

I woke up the next morning, a little groggy. I messaged Britney Spears to come visit me. I didn't realize I had a crush on her but apparently when you're powerful and famous I figured I may as well give it a shot. The next morning, she didn't come as I was expecting, so I was disappointed. *There must be some sort of problem getting here. Perhaps everyone is trying to fly in to my area and there are some major transportation issues as a result.* After breakfast, the nurses had me go talk to another patient there, or at least brought me into a room where he was. I believed they brought me there specifically to try to communicate with him. He was old, probably in his mid 60's, rocking back and forth, not speaking. I asked him if he heard ghosts too. He didn't respond. I tried communicating with him through telepathy, but it was if he wasn't there in his head to me. *This guy must be scared senseless*, I thought. *Perhaps he saw too many ghosts.* I really wanted to communicate with this old man, he probably had a lot going on in his head that could help me clarify what was happening to me. I gave up and went back to my room. Eventually I was moved to another part of the hospital, where more patients were staying. They even hung out and had lunch together. *Interesting, this must be the upper echelon of freaks at this place.*

At this new area, I was able to walk around, there were things to do. A nurse/male aid or someone came in who was about 6'4 350 lbs. When I gained a little more freedom, I realized just how much of my freedom was taken initially and this maddened me. I was irritated for being kept and began yelling and cussing at everyone and told them I was getting out of here now, it was time for me to go. They really pay a whole lot of attention to me it seemed, which was almost incredulous. Don't you people see how pissed off I am? Apparently not, so I decided to take a hostage. I grabbed the first person I saw and it turned out to be the big guy, he was the closest and he was also the strongest. It didn't matter, when you get that angry, something snaps and thinking is overpowered by that emotion. This is the same emotion that kills and hates people. Not controlled anger, but all-out rage. I put him in full nelson and we scuffled all the way across the floor to the other side of the room and fell. The next thing I knew there was about 4 or 5 people on top of me. One of them was a pretty nurse looking at me with a worried yet sorrowful look and I calmed down immediately when I gazed into her eyes. I became motionless which allowed them to lift me up and take me to a bed. They strapped me up to the bed with restraints then injected me with something. I then proceeded to talk to Brittany Spears with my ESP and tried set up a date with her. Before I knew it I was fast asleep.

I woke up the next morning still restrained to my bed. I didn't know why that was, forgetting completely all about the night prior. Perhaps it was too hard for my mind to remember and I blocked it out. Regardless, apparently these people think I'm dangerous. *They have no idea though*, I thought. *This is going to be epic.* I jerked violently, trying to free myself from these ridiculous leather straps. *Surely I am powerful enough to break out of here and tear this whole building down.* I failed miserably, and I saw red marks from the straps on my wrists. I must be weak still, after all this new found power of mine probably still has to grow. I began reasoning that I had this power due to some divine nature. *Am I the Messiah? Am I the antichrist?* I switched back and forth believing I was both, which in hindsight which one I was at the time depended upon the mood I was in.

I don't remember how long I stayed at St. Margaret's. I don't remember when they let me out of the restraints. I do remember looking out the window some days and watching the wind sway the tree branches and was able to translate the movement of the branches into the English Language again. I was back in the room with all the other patients again. As I gazed outside while the others ate their lunch, I noticed the trees and plants had been talking to each other... great. *I wonder if they're talking about me? Obviously they are.* This is not good, Mother Nature might possibly be plotting against me now. Well, in any case, there was another patient there that I needed to keep tabs on now. He didn't talk much and I learned his name was Adam from the nurses calling to him. I thought He was the original Biblical Adam, a reincarnation of the first human. I also assumed he was in the military, I don't know why. These thoughts dropped into my mind and became reality, no reasoning required when you're in this state of mind. Then I noticed my name was on a dry erase board with the other patients staying there. It had some check marks here and there, for what I wasn't sure. It seemed to be an aid for the nurses. My name, being Chris, but the board said Christ. This is either another coincidence or I hallucinated the T at the end of my name. *Are these people messing with me*? DO they think I think I'm Christ? *I guess so*, so I erased it. (Maybe they misspelled my name? I still don't know to this day). Apparently the medicine they were giving me was doing something. I was no longer interested in playing the role of the Messiah, or the Anti-Christ. I realized slightly that I must have been acting a little crazy, which is why I was there. Whatever they gave me was reducing the mania, but I still wasn't entirely back to normal.

The next day, we had a group meeting they wanted me to go to. I was starting to feel a little better as the meds were kicking in I think, whatever it was they were injecting in me. They had me do a collage. I put together a very deep collage in a few minutes from magazines... Some people were looking at me impressively including the worker there. The girl next to me kept batting her eyelashes. Then I noticed the male nurse sitting down across the table from me had a cast around his wrist. Then I noticed it was the guy who I tried to take hostage my first day. I felt like an idiot and the girl next to me passed me a note with a rose on it from one of her magazines with her number. It turns out she was bipolar too. I didn't know what was wrong with me at the time. I didn't even really grasp where I was either, who I was, or what I was doing there. I was just there, going through this time and space on autopilot. I was released that day. I guess it was around three to four days after I was admitted after punching the guy in the street corner, things moved very quickly for me there, perhaps due to my lack of insurance. My parents came and picked me up and lectured me on my drug use. I told them I guess I smoked something laced with PCP or something, only I didn't know it. I didn't know what was happening to me, and that was the best explanation I could come up with. Mental Illness never hit me as a possibility. I think that's what everyone else thought too, the symptoms I had were of some weird drug I took. The case was closed in my mind. I was released from the hospital after I started gaining some clarity and with the goal of going back to work.

Chapter 6

I went back to my job showing them the hospital papers. I hadn't called off any of the days I was missing. Not surprisingly, they didn't let me come back. Back into depression I went. I blamed them in my mind for discriminating against me due to a medical condition, but I took it no further, after all, I didn't call and show up on them for an entire week. As I stayed at home, my parents directed me to my next assignment which was outpatient therapy. I went along, all while taking steady doses of medicine that was initially prescribed to me upon my release. When they started me on the outpatient therapy program, I never saw anything like it. I tell you, the people who went to this place were nothing like me. They were all immature for being in their early 20's or older and had some pretty messed up directionless lives. I was functioning semi-normal at that point; the medicine was continually improving my mental health. I forgot really about all that happened to me, as I placed it in the back of my mind and chalked it up to some unknown hallucinogen that I took. I was taking it one day at a time. The outpatient program had arranged transportation for me picked me up on a bus every day. I went along, slightly begrudgingly. This seemed somewhat like school, which was 8-2:30 every week day. I really didn't like the whole set up. Anyways, there were quite some characters at this place. I felt a little humiliated, being treated essentially like child in grade school, but I persisted on. I was a little curious as well and had nothing better to do anyways. This turned out to be beneficial in the long run to me as I realized there were a lot of other people that were pretty messed up in their head out there. My therapists seemed impressed by my intellectual abilities, which made me think this place isn't for me. There are worse off people here. After some time of doing therapy, I worked on getting it to stop. Eventually I was able to visit a psychologist twice a week instead of attending therapy every day.

I ended up calling the phone number on the rose from the magazine and we went out a few times. She invited me to a party, which I accepted casually.   I drove about a half hour to meet up with her at her friends house and I ended up drinking around 3-4 beers. She got really mad at me for some reason and I suspected it was because I was drinking, as she knew I shouldn't be since we were both on medication after our release from the mental ward. *She seems to have her head on straight, she doesn't seem to be the kind of girl for me.* I was in no mood for some sort of uppity lifestyle at this point. At this party I was still slightly in my manic state, it seemed like I was just released from the hospital where I met her, but I wasn't acting out to anyone previously and just going with the flow, until I came here to this party. I remember having ESP again at the party, hearing people's thoughts. It didn't get me paranoid as we were all having a good time, but I didn't reason correctly and think these were hallucinations. Something about this ability made me want to keep it, it was exciting and accepting that it was all just my own delusion wasn't something I was up for yet.   While hanging out and socializing a bit, I realized something I said upset the girl I was with. I believe I was acting as if I was important, this all too familiar feeling of grandiosity was coming back at me with this consumption of alcohol *and it felt good*. Something I said angered her and she left. I didn't really care too much, *that was that*, I thought. I didn't know anyone there so I left too. I acted weird there, I don't remember what I did, but in hindsight I do know I shouldn't have been drinking. Part of me at the time knew I wasn't mentally healthy, the other part of me was still leaning towards psychosis. Thankfully, I ended up doing nothing else and arrived safely back at home.

After I was released from my first hospital stay and began outpatient therapy, I remember believing that I could communicate with anyone I was seeing on TV. I have since found out that this is pretty common, I wonder why? Anyways, television became pretty enjoyable at that point and I continued practicing my ESP powers through watching television. I preferred live television so I that I could communicate in real time with whomever was on TV, such as the news or sports. Then it started happening with taped broadcasts, of movies that were 10 and 20 years old. I thought I was supernatural and had the ability to somehow communicate through time as long as I was concentrating on it. This was happening with the music that I listened to as the lyrics seemed to be directly talking to me personally. I began thinking this is happening because it's the end of the world and I was a supernatural force, but I couldn't quite figure out what I was yet. I remember watching a tennis game and they showed a picture of the sky, it was ominously cloudy except a beautiful hole in a spot over the tennis court that let the sunshine come down. I thought it was because I was watching them from above, through a "God's eye" view. I thought I could improve the players' performances by using my mind. I would make them hit the ball extra hard if I concentrated on it. Everyone at the stadium that I saw on TV knew what was going on, they had the terrible notion pop into their minds as well through telepathy that some guy with divine powers was watching TV from his home communicating with ESP to everyone and manipulating the game. They were all in awe, all because of me. However my parents were avoiding talking about these miraculous powers of mine as they were my parents and that's how they were supposed to act. *They can't let me get a big head, of course.* I loved watching TV at that time. I remember watching the WNBA and communicating to the women on the court that whoever played the best would get to be one of my wives, then I started seeing them all play harder to compete for my love. Yup it was great. At this point they replied back and asked who I was; it occurred to me that I must be God. I started crying while watching this game and mentally started communicating to the world that God had came here to find a wife and the world was going to end but we'd all go to Heaven for living in the last days. *Yup, God's here and it's time to party!* Get the wedding preparations under way, God's getting married! The nonsense of this is completely embarrassing today, but my belief that I was God was fun nonetheless. To believe fully, that I held all the power of an almighty being and was just beginning to learn of my abilities was a joy only an insane person could experience.

Chapter 7

I was still attending my therapy during this time. It seemed the mania would fluctuate a bit, sometimes it would barely be present and other times it would be pretty heavy. When it was barely present I was almost thinking normal, but when it came back I was utterly psychotic. Another weekend comes by and I turned on the TV once again, as it was my way as God to communicate to people. I could manipulate however way I wanted. Sometimes I got confused but figured out logical explanations to myself as to why the person on the TV screen didn't do as I asked, even if it was Clint Eastwood performing in some Spaghetti Western 30 years earlier. I remember one Saturday turning on a White Sox game. The crowd started chanting my name as they knew I tuned in. I hated the White Sox, as I was a Cubs fan. They are eternal rivals in this two team city. The White Sox were playing in Chicago at the time in what was known as the "Crosstown Classic" It was happening only about 40 minutes away from me. I started talking trash to the White Sox pitcher to try to get him to mess up. During this period of time I was getting the notion that all the men in the world were against me because I was so powerful, and I also had gained the affection of all the women, creating some intense jealousy. *It doesn't matter, I'm God.* Even the White Sox opposing team, my team the Cubs, didn't want me to help them win their game. *All due to jealousy.* I started getting angry and engaged in a telepathic duel with the baseball player on television. When the camera crew focused on close ups of the player, I would see he would grin at me, or communicate through some other facial expression. All this was proof to me that we were communicating with our minds. I then threatened the pitcher that I was going to come up there to Comisky Park, because he seemed a little too cocky on television, during our communication. They showed a live shot of him and he mouthed the words "do it" to me. I knew that he meant to say that to me. Furious, I got dressed and I started thinking what I was going to do. *This guy's going to pay for that.* I drove up to Comisky and parked outside the park. The game just ended and the Sox won. I kept my word and made my appearance. I just sat there communicating with everyone who walked by. They knew I was there, that I was God, and that we were all going to Heaven so they were happy to see me. (The real reason is they were happy the Sox won). This changed my mood and I was no longer angry with the player who just challenged me on national television. I sat there in my parked car for a half hour or so, communicating with the fans there. Whether they saw me or not and walked passed while not acknowledging me didn't matter. *We all have to play it cool, you know we can't create pandemonium just because of my presence*. My mood was happy now and I carried on with one of my aimless driving sprees, gravitating in the general direction back to my house. Not only was all the music I was listening to directly talking to me (whether through time or not), but I was still talking to the world in my head. Good times, I tell you. *I'm God on Earth and I have ESP, all the women want me, the guys kind of despise me for that but hey, we're all going to Heaven and we're going to party until we do!* I ended up getting lost on my way home as I was taking a route I never did before.

I was running out of gas I had no money and started getting a little worried. I tried to grasp my bearings but it seemed every time I turned the sun would always be on my left side. I thought something was wrong, if this is happening I can't be God. I started freaking out and went to a gas station to ask for directions. I saw a cop on the road and ran up to him. I asked him how to get to Indiana, as that's where I lived. He looked at me a little weird and told me the directions. A little relieved I got in my car and took off in the right direction. I was really running low on gas... I remembered everything should be free for me but I decided since I started thinking I wasn't God anymore that people wouldn't give me free gas. I scraped together some pennies and put in less than a dollar and I ended up finding my way home. I was getting angry that this day turned out to be a disaster. *How could these people make me pay for my own gas?* I ended up going to sleep, because the next thing I remember is that I woke up to the voice of President Bush and one of his female aids communicating to me that I was a threat to his presidency and he would not stand for this crap that I was pulling with my telepathic powers. I felt as if our telepathic conversation was being recorded and the entire Defense Department was listening in as well. Then his female aid started rattling off all these things about me, where I lived, where I went to school, when I graduated. I started thinking, *damn it,* they know who and where I am *and* my life history. I started getting angry, I was feeling great, but something was brewing within me, something dark and not within my control. I would see later one of the most vivid hallucinations I can remember, that if anyone saw and heard this, they surely would go mad just from experiencing it if they believed it to be true.

I had therapy that day. I got up, ceased my ESP and got ready. I was going with my Mom, I was driving. On the way up there I realized that since so many people were against me, that I wasn't God, I was the Antichrist. *If the president isn't on my side, there must be something he knows that I don't.* That explains it, he knows I have a weakness. This also means that it was the end of the world, I was doomed to go to hell, but I was going to rule earth eventually. (I went to 13 years of Catholic schooling, I'm certain my religious background played a large role with my delusions.) On the drive up there, I turned to my mom and said "I wasn't really "born", was I. She said of course I was and seemed shocked for me asking a silly question such as that. She was in denial I thought. So... my Mom was impregnated by the devil. That explains why she had me at such an old age (she was 45). It all made sense now, the special powers, yet not the full almighty powers. I was doomed to burn... A little angry, excited, I then declared to the world that I was the Antichrist through telepathy. A sense of dread fell over the world as I mentally communicated this. I felt the impending doom; it was so real that I could've pissed my pants. I noticed a truck passing by in the oncoming traffic with a German Shepherd looking out the window. The German Shepherd opened his mouth and said "He's good", but in a very calm, odd, but soothing deep voice. Somewhat like the dog Brian, on "Family Guy". It was stunning to see a dog actually talk to me, the feeling I felt is certainly indescribable. In retrospect, it actually felt as if it were a mix of a panic attack and a lunatic high. I realized the apocalypse was going to bring all sorts of surprises. As I drove on, I pondered about what this dog just said to me as it drove by. He wasn't saying "I was good" as in not evil, but he was saying I was good on my declaration that I was the antichrist. I don't know how I figured this out, but this was my conclusion. *So it was true, I was the antichrist, the talking German Shepherd who just drove by confirmed it.* The panic and mania of this hallucination fueled my psychotic fervor to a climax and here we are on my way to therapy. The dread of being the spawn of Satan was too much for me to handle. The talking German Shepherd, the announcement that I was the Anti-Christ and the terrifying panic of the entire situation flowed through me. My mind was racing. I was doomed to burn in hell for being the Anti-Christ and now I have nothing left to lose. *At least the next 7 years or so will be enjoyable.*

I assure you I have no recollection of the rest of the drive there as the dog talking to me was utterly blowing my mind, causing my thoughts to race more ferociously and out of control than ever before. Once you see and here a dog talk to you, anything can happen. I believe I spoke to the President again during our drive, threatening him with my unholy powers. Either somehow we made it to counseling center without killing anyone. Convinced I was the antichrist I started getting scared. I remember thinking that I was the biggest son of a bitch that ever lived and I was scared of even myself. I believed everyone knew I was the antichrist too. I walked up to the patients hanging around outside and started asking people for cigarettes to bum, as I was all out. I was being nice because I didn't want anyone to start crying or anything, after all I was practically all powerful until Jesus arrived. Not only was I so powerful, I was crazy. I knew I was crazy in this aspect, because I was the antichrist. When I finished my cigarette, I asked for another one and then another one. Everyone was gone, I figured they don't want to hang around Satan himself, so I started asking the workers. They led me to a doctor who handed me a cigarette. I wasn't aware what was going on, but I was nervous and just couldn't control myself anymore. All of it was too much to take in. I believed my mom was talking to one of my therapists and I was getting upset about this, because I was the Antichrist, I thought she should be talking to me. *Therapy can't save me now, I'm far beyond saved.* I then opened up communication to George Bush again. Remembering this morning's discussion I was now armed with the new found realization of who I really was. I was Satan incarnate , prince of Darkness and I was doomed to burn for eternity. Somebody's going to pay for this.   The very fact that people wouldn't acknowledge my un-holiness in verbal speech was infuriating. Only telepathically would people discuss my status and our current situation of residing in the end of days. I told President Bush that I was going up to Chicago *right now* and I'm going to terrorize the city if he didn't make an announcement of some sort that would make everyone begin to recognize my power in public. At that moment, in a split second, I proceed to run out the clinic. I was on a mission to get this accomplished immediately. My mom and a doctor watching me didn't have a chance to stop me as I burst through the front doors outside. I got in my truck, turned the ignition and sped off and enjoyed this new found freedom of being alone as I felt enslaved driving with my mother to this "place". Everything seemed like a meager systematic method of confinement, some sort of sideshow to keep me busy and away from my real job, conquering the known universe. I certainly don't think they gave it their all to contain me, after all, the more they tip me off with increasing the security, they may make me realize that they just how dangerous I really was. If I knew how dangerous they thought I was, then they would know that I knew I was on to them. That wouldn't be good for me. Little did they know, I was well ahead of this game. My thoughts were scattered and fragmented. My actions based on whatever delusions and voices that popped into my head. I was completely out of control.

I was a mad, angry and thirsty, Satan. I was speeding, going through red lights, driving like a cop in a high speed chase. I flew around people in the wrong lane and was veering cars off the road. I came to a construction site where there was about a 3' deep crater about 30' long taking up the whole width of the road, it was clearly impassable for mere mortals. I started driving down the huge sinkhole and heard a deafening thud followed by a scraping noise. *Well my truck certainly isn't immortal.* Worried that my vehicle couldn't handle this, I put it in reverse and got out of there. I decided to leave Chicago alone at this point, and thought about my Mom who I just left there with no way home. *Yes I'm Satan, but I still have a mother and I just abandoned her.* I went back and she said, "thank God you're back." Still in my character of being the antichrist, a therapist came over and started talking to me. I asked for another cigarette and we stepped outside. I started crying and she began praying for me. The ambulance came and I got in quite peacefully. For some reason I felt that I needed to go in, just to get away from the stress of this apocalyptic world. I was on my way to St. Catherine Hospital in Whiting, Indiana.

Chapter 8

At the mental ward I came to the conclusion that the apocalypse had already happened and everyone I saw was already dead. I was in a certain hell, whether it was temporary until final sentencing or permanent, I did not know. The other patients there were ghosts, walking around in a daze. They seemed like lost souls trapped in purgatory. The workers there were just doing the work of God, but they weren't alive either. *These nurses are Possibly angels*. I started imagining how things were outside of the place that I was in. I looked at the windows and saw people walking around the neighborhood. *They're dead too,* I thought. While looking at the lost souls in the room around me, I started giving people alternate biblical identities. Adam was there again, so was Joseph this time. We were all there stuck in a hellish limbo, and it was my entire fault, I was the antichrist. I didn't speak to anybody, I was too exhausted.

During my time there, which was over a week, a lot of things happened and a lot of it is very blurry. I remember lying in bed, and in my mind images of earth from beginning to end swept through my head. It started with earth volcanic activity and pressed forward millions of years until there was life... I then realized since the apocalypse came that I was replaying the history of the universe in my head, as a "this is your life" episode, but it was with the universe. The images were fast and vivid. I didn't know what was happening. There were many voices now, they were loud and chatty. At some points it was like the crowd at a sporting event. I realized all the now dead people in the world were watching the replay of the universe with me and they were enjoying the show. I guess this is what happens at the end of time, we get to see how it all went down. *Cool.* I got up from bed and stepped out into the hallway, the voices immediately disappeared. This was terrifying because I didn't know where everyone went. I walked back into the room and the voices came back. I peaked my head out saw some dead people there walking and the voices disappeared again. This happened a few times... I began kicking the windows of my room as hard as I could. Nothing happened, it was some sort of indestructible plexi-glass. I pondered what would happen if I snapped everybody's neck here, after all they were already dead. I didn't think that would be too effective and it might get a little messy anyways. Throughout my time here I was drifting in and out of hallucinations and sheer madness.

One day during my stay the nurses called me up to the front office of the mental ward. My parents were here! I was so happy to see them. We went into a room and sat down with a doctor. They began talking to each other but I couldn't hear or understand anything they said because the voices were many and quite loud at this time. I tried focusing but couldn't. At this time I had been on some anti-psychotics for an unknown number of days. I still believed I was the antichrist and had telepathic powers, however, but it didn't carry over to everyone else. I mentioned that there was too much going on right now in my head and that I couldn't concentrate and apologized for it. I really wanted to have a conversation with my parents, but I couldn't with all the voices going on in my head. I don't even know exactly what the meeting was about. Looking back on this now I'm sure I may have looked catatonic, but I was completely aware and overwhelmed by the voices in my head. Soon enough, my parents left, which saddened me greatly, because I was too incapable of having a meaningful conversation with them. I walked slowly back into that hallway of hell which I currently resided and went to sleep.

Chapter 9

Days came and gone. I was still taking my medicine every day and having my blood checked every morning for my Lithium levels. I began to play games at the hospital with other patients and socializing a bit more. It was some number game I never played it before, but I remember I matched up the numbers 666 with my cards. I looked at everyone to see if anyone would freak out about me getting that number. *Everyone's cool*, so I carried on playing. I kept seeing odd number formations in the game we were playing, it was almost as if I was autistic at the time and having the ability to pick out codes and hidden messages. I never experienced anything like this in a mentally healthy state of mind. The game ended with nobody winning, which was the result of everyone's lack of focus. Perhaps they too were in some bad shape. I didn't know, I was more concerned with myself and my own issues at the time. I wasn't exactly sure what happened to me then, but about the time I played the game I remember having the mindset of being a little more self-aware that I may be mentally ill, but absolutely did not grasp this entirely. I remember watching a movie there. It was Tomb Raider. I realized that this movie was showing me what I would have to do later. I studied it. This someone was to prepare me for what I must overcome. By the end of it, the movie got so ridiculous that it seemed too impossible to be actually part of my life. Perhaps the medicine was kicking in even more. Closer, inch by inch, to sanity I transcended.

I remember hitting the call button a lot. The nurses eventually began to ignore me. There was this crazy girl that kept smiling and pointing her elbow at me. I figured she liked me but why was she pointing her elbows at me constantly? She was very weird, I was glad I wasn't as weird as her, I was thinking. But soon enough, I began skipping around the ward then started sliding on my socks on the laminate flooring. I was getting a little stir crazy, on top of being quite crazy aside from that. After days and days of being in there, I started feeling that I was going to be there forever. Not realizing how long I've been there and not seeing any hope in getting out, I once again went to my room and began kicking the plastic cover over my window so I could escape. It didn't work as it just bounced me back. I thought about stabbing my neck with a pencil. I guess at this time I didn't think it was the apocalypse. I heard a loud drilling noise. I got happy about that because I then began believing the US military was there drilling out the doors to get me the hell out of there. I later talked to the doctor there, apparently it was a meeting on whether I should be released or not. One of the questions she asked me was if I had any suicidal or homicidal thoughts. Of course I had homicidal and suicidal thoughts, doesn't everybody? I know better. "No", I replied. Towards my end of the stay they ended up moving me to the less secure part of the mental ward. It was nicer and we could watch TV all day. The lithium was kicking in I guess. I didn't like the blood being withdrew every morning to check my lithium levels because both of my arms were a bruised mess. I began asking the nurses at least twice a day when I could go home. I thought they were out to get me and that they were doing everything they could to screw me over there, to keep me as long as possible. I planned on calling a lawyer, got a phone book at took some phone numbers from it. I ended up never making a call. I spent the rest of my time reading the Bible a bit, trying to figure out my destiny. I ended up giving a call to a local Catholic Church and asked to speak to a Priest. Luckily, he was available and I asked some questions about what some things meant in the Bible, such as what is the difference between the son of God and Son of Man, as mentioned in various bible verses. I don't remember really what I was thinking at this point or why I was asking those questions. I remember one of my friends and a girl acquaintance from my high school visited me. At this time I was doing much better and they didn't understand why I had to be there. I really didn't know why I was there either at the time, as I didn't think about it. I was just somewhat relieved that I was still accepted socially somewhat. Soon after being transferred to the minimum security section of the mental ward, the day came when I was being released. I had talked to my parents about it and was ecstatic to be able to get out of there. I had no thoughts of being Satan, or the apocalypse, or anything else. Getting out of the hospital and getting some fresh air was all that was on my mind and I'm sure I seemed to be quite improved from when I first arrived. As I walked out of the hospital, it was beautiful, I remember. The air, the sun, the sky, something we all take for granted every day in our normal lives. I assure you, there are so many who would feel like they won the lottery if they just were able to step outside, something most of us take for granted every day. Nothing is as valuable to you as being able to step outside, when you simply are deprived of it for weeks or longer.

Chapter 10

After this event, I gradually spent more time in therapy, taking medicine and attending more therapy. The medicine I had was working, but I will still a few screws loose. I was getting sick from the medicine, spacing-out and drooling on myself. This was common due to the intense dosage of medications. I was taking Risperdal, lithium, and something else that I don't remember the name of. I complained to my mother that the medicine was making me sick. It felt as if I had nausea in my brain, the only way I could explain it to her. She didn't seem to understand that. I remember wasting my days away after being released from St. Catherine's mental ward. I resorted back to watching TV, having no money and not doing much at all except slowly recovering mentally, but not completely. I didn't really contemplate all that much on what had happened to me. I took for granted that once again I did some bad drugs and had a bad trip, but that doesn't really make a whole lot of sense since the whole mess lasted so long and I didn't even take any drugs that would cause that. Perhaps I was in denial about my situation. I wanted a way to get out of outpatient therapy and also wanted to go back to college. Going to college provided me with this option as I didn't have many other options available. My recovery took a whole summer and signed up at the local community college on one of the last days possible. I also got a part time job doing telemarketing while in school. I particularly remember my Communications II class it was the most fun. We had to prepare speeches and it was just a fun class overall for me. I didn't talk much to people there; I always wore a hoodie and looked like a skater punk all the time. Every time I looked at this girl in my class she would always get red... One day I got a haircut and she said she liked my hair and I said thanks. A few classes later I was the last student to leave because I was talking to the teacher, I walked out to the hallway and the girl was there waiting for me. She wore a skirt that day and was looking good. I never really talked to her but she just stood there waiting for me to get out of class. She asked me a couple questions about our assignment I think. We ended up talking about ourselves and I ended up asking her to go shoot some pool with me and one of my friends that I met in outpatient therapy. She said sure, gave me her number and that was that. I was on my meds and doing ok, and I remembered what I had gone through the months before. I was going to school full time again, working part time, and still doing some outpatient therapy when I felt like it. Things were looking much better for me, better than they had in the past year or so. For whatever reason, this girl was totally into me. I don't think we really didn't consider it a date since we were just playing pool but she had other things in mind I found out later. I brought my friend who ended up bringing another guy from outpatient, who was a complete *nerd*. He was 22 years old and loved "Pokemon". He was hilarious to talk to though because he was so nerdy. This guy was obviously something else. I didn't mind and thought it would be funny to have him hang out. I picked her up and the four of us went to play pool. She was looking hot again this night. We played some pool and my friend started hitting on her. I was casual and let things ride. I ended up poking her in her crotch with my pool stick by accident while shooting, *a sign of things to come.* I didn't really hit on her while playing pool though, but I said I was sorry and she said it was fine and smiled. We ended up going to the park where I used to hang out and drink with friends because it was a little secluded. Billy, the nerd, never drank a beer before so we talked him into it. I told him its time for you to become a man. He enjoyed his beer and we started messing with him. There was an outhouse there and Megan, the girl, told him that's where she lived sometimes. He believed it and started asking all these questions about it. He then proceeded to puke all over the place. *These people I hang out with are morons.* It was getting cold outside and I made my first move on her and started rubbing her back to warm her up. Later I found out that she didn't recognize this as flirting and was tired of my other friend hitting on her the whole time. Things were looking promising, at least for me and this new girl I met. Being mentally healthy I was able to pursue another interest that the mania had put on hold, *women.*

A few days later I called her and asked her if she wanted to go grab something to eat. We went to Pizza Hut, it was right by her house. I got a call from my friend and he said he was having a party at his house, I asked if she wanted to go and she did, so we left. When we got there my friend started gave her a nice compliment about her beauty as we walked in. We had a few beers and then I noticed my friend holding Megan from behind as they walked up the stairs and she looked behind her kind of surprised. *Alright, I had enough of this.* I brought her here and she's mine. I made my moves and we kissed for the first time and we stayed side by side the rest of the party. From then on I pursued her until she became mine, she is with me to this day.

That college year went well. I really eased up on drug use since I entered a relationship with Megan, my girlfriend. Months into our relationship we fell in love and both told each other this. We hung out every day after school until we left for our jobs. Then after work we hung out if we could. We spent Holidays at each others families and things were going well. I told her about my past experience with the mania, she didn't care she loved me for who I was now. Another school year began and she went to an art school downtown Chicago, I did another semester at the community college. Frustrated by my grades in math I stopped attending my classes. I also stopped taking my meds regularly at some point. This was just because I was doing so well, I felt as if I didn't need them anymore. I was also still in denial about my mental health. I quit school and started looking for a good job so I could move out. I applied to get disability, but they declined me. I had no other choice but to look for a job. I ended up sending résumé's everywhere again. A guy called back who worked downtown Chicago and asked me to bring some writing samples. I wasn't sure what the job was for and was confused why the writing samples were requested. I wore my best shoes and black suit and headed up for the interview downtown. The building was huge and it was in the business district. I had some decent works experience on my resume from the jobs before my mania, and I had elaborated on my length of stay at my past job that I got fired from. This allowed me to only apply for management positions. The owner looked at my resume and said I had some pretty good skills for such an age. He showed me the stack of résumé's he received so far, he said it was in the hundreds and said I had the best written resume out of all of them. I wrote it myself so that felt good to me. It turns out the job was to run a resume writing office solo in another location. He was the best and one of the only resume writers in Chicago. I would be in an office in a business building similar to his, and would basically run the show. He would do the advertising and I would handle calls and arrange appointments for me to discuss how I would handle their resumes. The minimum fee was $50 for a basic resume, all the way up to the thousand dollar mark, or whatever I could get away with charging. Training began and he showed me the ropes, which would last about a month. I was to get paid a salary and commission for the office that I was going to be in. I was excited and Megan was very happy for me. Everything was going so good for me, maybe I felt a little too good, because the mania began kicking in again. It was a lose/lose situation. If I was happy I became manic off my meds, if I was having a downslide, deep depression was on the horizon. I had been under the impression that if the psychotic episodes happened again I would be able to recognize it ,which is one of the reasons why I went off the meds, but once it starts you can't. It just spirals out of control. It grabs ahold of you and blinds you to everything sane and rational.

I remember walking around my workplace and feeling supernatural. I was in a hallway and I breathed in and out and I saw the walls move with every breathe I took. I was like *Neo*, from the Matrix, as he envisioned Agent Smith at the end of the movie. I was feeling euphoric and all so powerful again.

The mania was getting more dangerous by the day, slowly building over the period of about a week or two. At work, occasionally the boss had me do some paperwork on his computer in the city. I saw a payroll file on it and I clicked it open. I searched for the salary history of the person who I was going to be taking over for. He was making $250 a week, which upset me, for this job I was expecting quite a bit more in compensation for this line of work yet I decided to hang in there for a bit. I remember cashing an old check one day. I walked into the bank and gave the teller my check. He mumbled something to me like "he's the Christ", begrudgingly. My check was for somewhere around $150.00 from what I could honestly remember. He handed me about $500 extra in one hundred dollar bills. I took the money, thanked him, he nodded and I left. I went shopping and bought some things, but I still had a lot of money left. To this day I have not figured out how exactly this happened, perhaps it is an incorrect memory, but I am quite certain I didn't make enough money to come out of that bank with the money I did. This made my situation a bit more bearable, at least in my mind.

One day on my way to work in Chicago and getting more manic by the minute, I got confused by missing some traffic signs. I wanted to turn left on to a street with traffic going in both directions. I never saw the do not turn left sign. I attempted my turn and little did I see that there was a traffic cop right in front of me. She stood in the way of my truck and told me to go straight instead. I was angry and I got out of my truck and talked to her. I didn't understand what she was saying for some reason but I ended up patting her on her shoulder and left. I drove off hurriedly. Before I knew it, a different cop pulled me over and arrested me. They gave me the reason that I was obstructing traffic, when I was confused about the traffic signs. As it turns out, I didn't have my license on me either, so they took me down to the station, I was under arrest for not having my license. While in the squad car, I either hallucinated or didn't, but I smelled alcohol on the arresting officers' breathe. After they released me at the station I headed straight for my job. He seemed pretty understanding and I told him I thought my arresting officer was drunk. He let me go to City Hall to file a complaint. When I got there nobody would help me out about filing a complaint. I told them to go get this officer off the road now since he's driving drunk. They said I had to call a certain phone number or go to this other office. This infuriated me, *I need answers and I need them now*. I yelled out as loud as I could in the Chicago City Hall "THIS CITY IS SO CORRUPT IT MAKES ME SICK!" Which ironically, it is corrupt of course, everyone knows that. I said it out of pure madness however. Nobody really reacted, perhaps this is a normal occurrence in Chicago's City Hall, I wouldn't know as I don't spend much time there these days. I stormed out of city hall looking around at the people as I left. Nobody laid eyes upon me while I exited. I headed to the location where I was directed to file my complaint. Upon arriving at this location they told me I couldn't file a complaint there. They gave me the run around and gave me a number I could call. *More bullshit*, I thought. *This city has me running a wild goose chase just to cover their asses.* The mania was driving me now. I didn't have a cell phone so I asked if I could use their phone and they said no. This pissed me off some more because there's still a drunk cop driving around as far as I'm concerned and nobody's doing a damn thing about it. Furious and even more manic now, I leave and start running to the next phone I could find. I walked around outside and run into a warehouse and tell a worker there I need to use the phone, there's an emergency. I call the number they gave me to report my suspicions. I guess I ended up giving them the address where I was calling from, because a few minutes later the cop I was calling to complain about showed up. *Son of a bitch! I can't believe I am calling the police to make a complaint about an officer and they send that officer to take the complaint.* He comes up to me and asked what was going on. I told him my suspicions and he denied it all. He was by himself, which freaked me out a little, because after all I was trying to get this guy in some serious trouble. I told him "it's ok I believe you." I was getting paranoid that he was going to throw me in jail out of spite. I said I was sorry for bothering him because I just wanted to get out of there and I didn't want any problems. I was manic, but I wasn't in the state of mind of being all powerful. I got in my car and drove away, thankful that I was able to avoid an incident. I later sent my boss a letter of resignation, telling him that he was a cheapskate. He read it in front of me and looked a little surprised. I had enough of Chicago at that time. Fortunately, I didn't get in any further trouble with the Chicago Police that day. I had a court date with them some weeks later and ended up having to pay a fine for driving without a license. *No big deal.* This time my father came with me. He as certainly concerned about my safety but he too had an anti-government mindset about him and he wanted to make sure the court did not try to screw me over. Being from an era where perhaps a father's presence might actually affect the outcome of the case. That is what he told me at least, he probably wanted to make sure though that I didn't get in any more trouble in Chicago, which after losing his son there, grew to hate that city more than any other. As expected, I had to pay a fine and was soon headed back home.

Chapter 11

Jobless again, the mania was growing now, overcoming me once more. Further and further I drifted off into madness, a realm I created had opened its doors to me and locked me in, with no recollection of the world I came from. How I got here was not a question that ever crossed my mind, all that mattered was, I was here, this is my world and my destiny lies ahead of me. I began writing on my black truck with soap to deliver messages, I really don't remember much. I wrote weird, crazy stuff about news events and more symbols. I know something I wrote stated "Crucify me upside down". I figured that was my destiny when it was all over with, when this wretched planet was laid waste by my unholy army that was inevitably to come. In the news, Libya had declared nuke free at that time and I loved it. I wrote on my truck that "Libya is saved". By saved, I meant, they were saved from my own destruction, not that I realized nobody would understand what I was talking about at all. That didn't matter, because everyone always knew who I was everywhere I went, in my own mind. I had a lot of symbols on my truck, such as crosses, the Jewish Star, the symbol for infinity, a crossed out Nazi symbol as if to say "No Nazi's". My messages on the back window of the cab would change on a regular basis. My truck was just covered with these things. I would drive around thinking I was God or the antichrist again and the music was talking to me. One day I wrote on it "God loves you". *God being me of course.* Somebody flipped me off. I blew them a kiss, in kind. It's a surprise not many people started trouble with me. To me though, it wasn't. *They should bow down before my very feet.*

On a random weekend night I went out with my sisters and Megan to a nice piano bar one day. They tell me I was talking crazy but I don't know what I said. We went home and I began reading the Bible with Megan. I read Revelations a lot because I started believing it was pertaining to me. I got to the part where the wine poured out after the angel killed all these people. I felt the taste of blood in my mouth as I read this. I asked Megan if she tasted it too and she nodded, she was obviously a little scared but was playing along at the time. I ended up going to another bar with just me and Megan. There I told her that when I died everyone else was going to too. I told her it was like I was the biggest nuclear bomb ever. We went to the book store Borders one day. She liked looking at a book of tattoos as she was an artist, she only has one herself. I never liked them. I told her that tattoos were evil, this ended up making her want to leave, which we did. On the drive home she said she thought tattoos were cool because they were kind of dangerous. I then said, "You want danger? Here you go." I floored it. She started crying and I was happy that I taught her a lesson. This whole time Megan knew I had relapsed. She loved me so much she wanted to be with me to help. She was telling my family everything that was going on with me. They were discussing what to do and in the process of arranging the help I so desperately needed.

I was driving to Chicago in the middle of night with my truck riddled with symbols written in soap. I couldn't sleep I was so manic. Things were getting bleak in my mind and the world was ending soon, once again. It seemed all my past psychotic breaks were being rolled into one continuous loop, and my moments of sanity were thrown right out the window. I wasn't eating much. One night I drove to Chicago and rolled my windows down. It was about 3 in the morning. The wind began talking to me as it rolled past my ears I translated it into English. I listened and obeyed the directions from it. It told me where to drive. It gusted particularly hard when it was angry, sort of like yelling at me. I obeyed diligently, sometimes narrowly missing my street altogether but taking hard evasive actions to maintain the course that the wind guided me on. I ended up vomiting out my truck window from being awake so long and from not eating much. I was physically exhausted and needed food. I went to a 24 hour McDonalds and asked for some water. They handed me my drink, I grasped it, and then I pointed at the dark green puke rolling down my door and said, "You see this? This is your sin." She gave me a disgusted, odd look. I drove off, thinking nothing of it. *Hmmm.. What else is going to happen tonight*, I thought. *Perhaps I should take up preaching.* It was about 6 in the morning and I was on my way back to Indiana after all night driving around. The voices were back in full force and so was my ESP. The sunrise was beautiful and the clouds had messages in them for me. I saw a Cross in the sky, hands held in prayer, and various other things. I thought Jesus was coming back and it would all be over soon. I was on the highway going about 70 when I started feeling faint. I pulled over to the shoulder, got out of my truck and collapsed in the grass. A State Trooper pulled behind me and I immediately got up. I was terrified I was going to jail. He asked if I was alright and I told him sometimes this happens to me and I get faint.   He then asked if I needed an escort and I said yes, that would be nice. He followed me until I got a few blocks from home and he pulled up to my side and I said thanks, I was relieved that I wasn't going to jail for something. Quick thinking led to him not questioning me further. I was drained and obviously not in a healthy state of mind.

During this time I was getting in a lot of arguments with my parents. For one I was gone all the time all hours of the night. All my money was being spent on gas and cigarettes and I wasn't even working.   I was a terrible pathetic person, looking back, however help was on the way. One day at home I just got out of the shower and was half naked drying myself. Cops came in the room and said to get dressed, I was leaving. I was confused and had no idea why. My parents weren't saying much. The police gave me a signed order by the Judge to admit me to the hospital. But I was fine I said, I've been fine for awhile. They didn't listen. I tried to get out of a stay at the hospital but they were admitting me no matter what. I should note also that at some point around this time I had broken up with Megan, I'm not sure when, it is a vague memory. It was probably before they came to my room to take me back to St. Catherine's hospital.

Chapter 12

I felt betrayed when I was in the mental ward the third time. I faked being sane as best I could. I faked taking the pills. I felt everyone was out to get me again. I was furious with my father for arranging my stay here. One of the doctors said I had pulled a knife out one day when I was arguing with them and threatened to slash my throat, which is why I was there. I remembered now, but told them it was just an argument and I was trying to display how angry I was. I was doing whatever I could to not take their pills as I thought they were poisoning me. It slowed me down, made me drowsy. It took away my entire personality. Being through this before, I plotted on getting out of there as soon as possible. I knew how to act and what to do, and I pulled it off. I faked it good enough to get released after three days. Once out I was furious but kept it to myself somewhat. I will still manic, plus anger. Not a good combination. When we got home I exploded in anger at my parents with a tirade of words. I was out of money and unable to do anything, tensions were high in the household. I'm not sure what they were thinking since I was just released, but I wouldn't give them time to react, aside from having my keys taken from me and being told I was not allowed to go anywhere. One thing for sure, the immediate future was not very promising.

Things were going to escalate very quickly, my intolerance of being controlled was coming to a head, as well as my mania.

The next morning, stolen keys in hand, I peeled my truck out of the driveway, angry that an attempt of my freedom had been made the night before. I had lost it again, completely psychotic now. I was feeling reckless due to having *won* this war with my parents and was in a mood to celebrate. As I turned up my music and drove on, the lyrics were guiding me. This was Nine Inch Nails – "Head like a hole, I got your soul!" I thought I had everyone's soul and I felt like God again. I went to the mall as everything for me was free. I had a red hoodie sweatshirt on that I had prepared nicely. It was marked with the symbols I put on my truck. It was anti Nazi, antichrist, 666, the Davidian Star, every religious symbol I could think of was on there. A lot of question marks were on there too, why I put them there I don't know, I was intrigued by the question mark symbol at that time. It was all written in black permanent marker. I walked into the mall looking like a madman. It was crowded as usual. I headed to get some more music to feed my mania. I walked into the CD store. I started snorting at everyone in there and grabbing CD's at random. I had about 10 of them. Even though I had hundreds of dollars in my pockets, I wasn't going to pay for them because they were free for me. People were looking at me and getting scared. The cashier yelled out "Be Gone Satan". I think she did at least. I looked at her held up the CD's I was taking to show her and growled at her on my way out. I calmly walked through the mall to get back to my truck. Mall security showed up and confronted me. I kept walking. They grabbed my arms from behind and tried to

handcuff me. They got one cuff on me and the scuffle began. I
didn't throw any punches, I just didn't let them handcuff me or
bring me to the floor. I had extraordinary strength at this time as
if I was possessed or on PCP. I was taller than both these guards
but they were meatier than me, yet they could not move my arms
at all no matter how hard they tried. I just kept them straight
down. One had my left arm one had my right arm. They were
using both their arms on my one arm and they couldn't get me
cuffed. This went on for quite some time and then I finally let
them cuff me because we weren't going anywhere fast. They had
me wait in this little office while they called the police to take me
to the jail. I thought nothing of why I was there or how my divine
will was being tampered with by these mere mortals. On the way
there I was cordial to the cop who came to pick up me. I talked
about his family and baseball and ordinary things. I was feeling
pretty good but my actions and thoughts were completely
unpredictable. Somehow after completely freaking out in the
mall just a few minutes earlier, I was able to have a completely
rational conversation with my arresting officer. *Madness, such a
fickle disease.*

The jail cell was a hellhole, with a blinding light constantly on
me. It looked like shit. There was a drunkard in the cell next to
me, and some kid who was there for a week or so. I started
messing with the drunken guys head. I began attempting to do
some voodoo magic or something, which I knew nothing about. I
looked at the blinding light, my eyes were closed just enough that
I could see through my eyelids and then an image appeared. It
was an old man, in a robe, standing on a black marble floor in

front of a beautiful pool of blue water at night. I didn't know what it was. I thought to myself if that was God that I just saw. It was quite possibly the most beautiful image I have ever perceived. When I realized how beautiful it was, I was worried that it would disappear. Unfortunately, it faded away. I stared as much as I could into the center of the bright bulb, hoping I could see the image in this rusty iron cage I was trapped in. I couldn't get it back no matter how hard I tried, all I could do was repeat in my memory the vision, which couldn't compare to the hallucination I just saw. Of course, during that incident, it was not a hallucination; it was a part of my role, as Messiah, or as antichrist, whichever it may be. At that time I was confused who I was supposed to be exactly but that didn't matter, what mattered was I was stuck in this cell and needed to get out.

I called my Dad and told him I needed to get bailed out. He got another family member to come and help pick me up from the jail. He was entirely concerned and furious. I had $400 in my pocket which confused everyone why I tried to steal a few CD's. I needed a little more to bail myself and dad came through. He wanted to drive me home, but I went home by myself. I was overbearing and demanding and left regardless. Nobody was telling me what to do, no matter what. My poor Dad, he was in his late 70's. This makes me want to cry thinking of what I did to him. I had put both my parents through hell and didn't realize it one bit.

The next morning my dad said I was absolutely not driving anywhere again. I knew he had other plans in mind as well. Of course, this infuriated me once again as I was not in any sort of rational state of mind. I ran out of the house with my keys and drove off once again. My father was not good at hiding and I knew all of his spots. Away I went, my parents, probably feeling hopeless, were the last thoughts on my mind now. I was tired of getting stuck in my plan of world domination. The loop of manic episodes melted together. I was in my crazy red hoodie again, with symbols written all over it. I was listening to some Wu Tang this morning as one of their CD's is apocalyptic in some ways. The plan was to take the cops on a high speed chase. I needed gas to do this. *Good, I'll steal it, even though it should be free, people aren't recognizing my power.* As I thought this, it just contributed to my anger. I headed to a gas station to fill up. I knew what I was doing, *taking what's mine.* I danced my way inside to the music. I had a good sound system and it was loud inside my truck, almost deafening. The symbols were all over me and my truck. I would have hated to have seen myself looking back on this. I handed the clerk an old navy credit card that was maxed out to use for my payment. I danced my goofy ass, yes literally danced, back out of there and drove off. For some reason I was in a good mood for taking the gas and believe me, I really don't dance well. Down the road ran into some traffic as I made my escape from the gas station. There were a lot of cars ahead of me and cars behind me at this red light. I noticed the flashing lights of a police car a few cars behind me. *Shit! I am not even on the expressway yet. This was it I am not going to get pulled over at a red light*, not in this state of mind. I bashed a few cars out of the way to make my escape and drove up a curb onto a grassy field to cut over to the next street. Then cops came out of every direction when I hit the road. I drove on casually, planning my moves. A cop pulled up to my side and mouthed the words "pull over now" to me. His face was full of anger. The music was and I was riding high on mania, I kept going. I suddenly floored it and turned left sharply, cutting off the cop who was on my left side. My truck began fishtailing violently as I made a tight turn down the residential street. I was aiming to go around the red light in which I was stopped at previously to get back on the road that will take me to the highway, *as well as 100 mph.* Suddenly, Cops appeared out of nowhere in front of me. I quickly surveyed the scene. There was a commercial style garage to my right in a large grassy field. There were train tracks ahead and the gates were blocked by cops. I had no other choice but to try to go over the railroad, where there is no road. I drove into the field to the right of me and tried to driver over the train tracks. Flooring it, the rails were too high when I passed over them and I ended up getting stuck. The body of my truck was teetering on the railroad tracks as the rails were too high for the wheels to touch the ground. I was wedged with my wheels in the air. I got out of the truck and put my hands in the air immediately as cops were running at me with their guns drawn. I got down on the ground with my hands behind my back and laid there for a second. The next thing I knew the barrel of a gun was jammed into my head and the cop yelling some curse words at me. Realizing I was just pistol whipped after submitting, I yelled out, *"Do you believe in God*?" They said nothing to me. One of the officers forced his knee on my head while I lay on the ground and proceeded to handcuff me. *They didn't need to use such force, I was motionless.* They lifted me up and pushed me on a cop car. Blood began pouring from my head onto the shiny white hood of the cities squad car. The pistol whip really did a number on me and soon I was on my way to jail.

Chapter 13

The city police station was nothing but a holding cell. I was able to calm down after this event while the officer wrote me up. I was in a small cage, fit for being held an hour or so. It looked like a locker, being that there wasn't any room to walk around in, just to sit there. I felt like I was in a bird cage. I began sitting there like a bird since I thought this. I began thinking I was a bird. *I was fucking gone.* The police acted like they saw this kind of nonsense all the time, and handled the paperwork for my transfer to county jail as if this type of reaction happens all the time. Reluctantly, I didn't start tweeting like a bird at least. I just perched my legs on the bench, rocking back and forth. It wasn't long until they got me out of there and took me into a squad car for a ride up to the county jail, which was about 30 minutes away. The ride there was enjoyable; it was peaceful for the most part and rather uneventful. After the uprising I just pulled off, it was time to just go with the flow for now. Upon entering the holding cell at County, I found myself with a few other criminals. Being very delusional I was wondering if I had to kill them or if they'd try to kill me. I was walking around the concrete blocks they had as seats as if it were a playground, but everyone was keeping to themselves. There was an intercom to call the guard and I began hitting it numerous times. The security guard I remember was getting very annoyed with me and I said sarcastically, "Are you *The One*?" Of course, however, I thought I was *"The One"* and I was simply making fun of him in my own mind. Shortly after they called me out and took me away for finger printing. Two guards escorted me into an elevator, I pointed out the necklace one of the guards was wearing. It looked like a Davidian Star only modified a bit as the top point of the star was rounded. I asked him what it meant and he said it was the star of Lucifer, the Davidian Star melted by the devil. I asked him if he "wanted to burn in hell". He didn't take too kindly to that question and soon enough I found myself in my solitary cell, but not only that, I had to strip down naked in there. The only thing I was provided to wear was an oversized paper towel about three feet long and two feet wide. I wrapped it around me like a Greek Toga. There was a concrete slab for a bed in the middle, with a metal hook on it. Fortunately I wasn't chained to it, but being nearly naked and locked in there was bad enough. I was confident, however that this cell would not be able to contain me. I ended up falling asleep after some time of manic thoughts listening and trying to make out my surroundings as much as possible. The next morning, breakfast was served through a slit. I had to come and get it myself. Completely naked I walked up as if I was the antichrist. I assumed they'd be terrified of me, seeing me in my true unholy form as it were, without any clothes. This went on a few days, when finally I was provided some clothes. They were comfortable. The cell was utterly boring, I had nothing but my own mad thoughts to keep me entertained, however that was more than enough. I was living my own sci-fi movie as if it were reality. I had a whole new world to explore, with some of the most dangerous people in the area around me. *I might be able to use this.*

I didn't realize it at the time but of course I was in the area of the jail where the "crazy" people go. I was on the floor with the other head cases. In the cell next to me I heard some loud banging of metal on metal. Someone was pretty upset it seemed as I began hearing cursing and yelling. His temper tantrum couldn't be ignored so I began peering out through the small window on my door. Suddenly water started seeping into my cell through the doorway. This guy had had managed to destroy his own toilet. *It seems he some talent.* Considering everything in the room is bolted down I thought this was quite the accomplishment. I stepped over the water and saw more of it that was pouring out into the hallway from his cell. Soon a few officers with a riot shield showed up. *This guy doesn't have a chance.* They hauled him out of there kicking and screaming. Who knows where they took him, *it couldn't be any worse than this place.* I went back to my concrete slab pondering what the other inmates were doing. *Nothing to do here but think.*

If I wasn't thinking, a lot of my time in the cell was spent blindfolding myself and memorizing my room. I was trying to sharpen my mind someway, to prepare for my release. I was highly manic and delusional still. One morning while washing myself up in the metal sink I found myself lost in the droplets of water that remained in the basin. I began peering into it as if I just uncovered the key to some existential crisis. The droplets of water intrigued me and I became lost in their form; I focused on one in particular and then suddenly it just disappeared on me. Shocked by this, I thought I just disintegrated the water with my mind. I did it again with another droplet and to my surprise, the same result! *The fucking water vanished,* I thought. I was able to eliminate many droplets of water by staring at them. *This talent is going to be very useful.* I kept practicing and it was quite enjoyable. I was working my way up to disintegrate the door in front of me. Yes, I was supernatural, I knew it! *All this trouble I have went through, the mental wards, and all the telepathic thoughts I had before did happen for a reason! I was the antichrist.* I wasn't able to shake this psychotic notion and I was once again living the life you only read about in comic books. Yet, something in me changed as I got bored with destroying water droplets. I was fickle and I lost focus, then I lost my power. I can't explain this in any other way today, except that it was all my hallucination. I still remember it as it clearly happened. Most hallucinations in hindsight I can remember as a hallucination, but not this. Nonetheless it powered my confidence in my supernatural abilities and when you're in jail; confidence is all you need. I was far too psychotic then to understand this, but this fueled my brazen interaction with the other inmates. I wasn't focusing on mental telepathy this much as the voices in my head weren't there anymore, but still had plenty of madness to keep me going.

After a couple weeks of remaining in solitary confinement each day, I was granted the luxury of having an hour outside of the cell. Finally I only had to spend 23 hours in that small hell hole. Each day during this time I was allowed to go to the community television room. There we can play cards, checkers, or watch television. I couldn't wait to get my eyes to the screen to view the unraveling apocalyptic world that surely was occurring outside. As I entered the television room, I noticed a few guys watching Laverne and Shirley or something absolutely unimportant and ridiculous. I couldn't believe these idiots would be watching something so inane that when I noticed they were distracted with their own socializing and after gaining some orientation to my new surroundings, I turned the channel immediately to the news and stood in front of it eager to see the world aflame. Unfortunately, things weren't progressing as I envisioned them. Normal news stories were however not a deterrent, as they were embellished in my mind to mean something exponentially greater in the grand scheme of my psychotic frame of reference that this was the apocalypse. Major traffic jams on the Dan Ryan expressway? *A massive unauthorized evacuation of course.* The media should certainly keep quiet about this, for the sake of containing the fear of my impending unholy wrath that will occur. Nothing, not even a fully normal functioning society with every day occurrences and tragedies was going to slight my understanding that this was the end of days. Reality was whatever my psychotic mind made it to be.

As the days passed I continually had my little challenge with the rest of the cell block about what to watch on television for the one hour a day. The television kept changing back to sitcoms, I kept changing it to the news. I noticed some people were getting annoyed however looking back, I'm sure they could see my mental state within. I am not a big intimidating guy at 6'2 180, very wiry, but I wasn't one to mess with, not in my state of mind at the time. I was capable of anything and I believed the inmates knew it. I somehow gained some respect there, with minimal social interaction. This is what it takes to gain acceptance in jail and it is just the opposite of what it takes to gain acceptance in society and I sure the hell had that going for me. There were however, some people that were never able to leave solitary confinement during my stay there. These were the ones that were considered murderers, as well as crazy. For me at that time, I was very lucky not to have been in that situation myself.

Time was going slow. While I may have spent a month and a half in the County Jail, it seemed to me like half of a year. As I was able to get out of my cell an hour a day, I peered through the windows of the cells around me as I walked down the hallway. I recognized someone in the cell next to me who had been in the news just prior to my incident. It was David Maust, who was recently jailed for raping and killing young boys, a relatively infamous person who made headlines with his crimes in the local paper and the Chicago Television stations. He wasn't let out at all and was entirely dismal looking. I found out years later he killed himself in that same jail, hanging himself by his sheets. I didn't think about him much when I was there as he was mostly out of sight, out of mind. That floor was filled with all types of people of the worst kind. At about this time, a lady began coming by every morning with pills. They were trying to poison me, I thought. They wanted to slow down my natural abilities. I knew what their plan was, to sedate me. I put it in my mouth, preparing to spit it out as I did previously at the mental wards. This didn't work this time, as it dissolved immediately when it hit my mouth. She asked me to open my mouth and asked me a question, making sure I had no choice but to swallow some. I did the best I could to spit out everything else once she had left. Every morning the lady showed up with medicine and she was definitely on to my attempts to not take it. She knew I didn't want the medicine and I did everything I could to not take it. It made me feel so different. It was a heavy dose of anti-psychotics, but that didn't mean anything to me, they were just trying to prevent my rise to power. After awhile I began to feel the effects of the pills, it began to make me feel like my blood was trying to come out of my body at times, something I've never felt before. The effect of this pill was extremely potent. I couldn't sleep because this was highly uncomfortable, my blood felt hot. I hated this medicine, but soon found myself complacent as every day I took it I couldn't help but ingest some of it. As time passed I gradually succumbed to their administered doses and stopped spitting out the medicine. I don't remember much of what occurred the next few weeks, but I soon had hope to be leaving jail as I was informed I would be transferred to my court hearing.

The day of my court appearance quickly came and I was ecstatic about the chance to see the outside world again. I was handcuffed and lead in the back of a van, the seating was very uncomfortable but I had a great view of the outside world again. I was with a few other inmates and the thought of escaping with them entered my mind, but I was so happy to be out of my cell, it quickly left. It was a hot day and we were headed about a half hour away, to the city of Hobart, for the incident in the shopping mall, in which I declared I was the one true God. I felt like Jesus, on trial for blasphemy. We parked, got out and I entered the courtroom and sat perfectly still, I was focusing on becoming a stone, on a whim. A fly found its way on my head, I didn't budge. I noticed the Judge's name was "Longer". Immediately I began wondering if this was some sort of changed last name to impress prospective mates through this subliminal assertion of his phallus size. *What a crock of shit*, I thought. The games these people play... and here he is a Judge, probably only because of his last name, at that. My thoughts were under the will of this maniacal disease that has overcame me. As the proceedings went on, I came to the conclusion that he was a fair guy, judging by the people that had to go before me. I plead guilty to the charges and was sentenced to community service and was able to be released in a few days. I was ecstatic and mildly manic. The medicine I had been taking was doing some good, but it wasn't enough time for me to lose the mania and psychotic thoughts. My parents were there and they comforted me greatly. I was able to say hello to them and was transferred shortly after back to my cell.

Chapter 14

The day of release was a happy one, I was looking forward to it for sometime, but I never knew when it was going to arrive. Suddenly I was called out of my cell, not knowing what was going on. I was then out of the door sooner than I thought. The sunlight of the jail lobby immediately enthralled me. My father was there waiting for me. When I walked out of the jail, the sun and breeze were so refreshing, that I couldn't be any happier. I got in the car and my dad was taking me to Ponderosa for a meal. I had lost weight from jail food and I was prepared to eat like an animal. During the drive to the restaurant, I ended up getting perturbed, for no reason. I was angry and I didn't know why. I remember watching all the cars driving around us and how they were all in such a hurry, yet I had just spent over a month doing absolutely nothing. The hustle and bustle of the world and my position in it made me realize everyone was getting themselves in a damn hurry for no good reason. Unfortunately, I wasn't able to look at it other than my own perspective, which was a calloused and shortsighted one. I ended up arguing with my father over it, it was unfortunate I would be in such a mood on this day that I was able to obtain freedom again. I felt like an ass and attempted to calm down. The food at the restaurant was extremely delicious. I couldn't ever remember eating a tastier meal. Believe

me, after eating jail food and losing weight because they just
don't serve you enough, going to McDonald's is just as good as
eating at a Zagat rated restaurant in downtown Chicago. Life was
great for me at that moment, considering where I had just been
the past two years. I was allowed to live back in with my parents.
The best was yet to come for me. I was coming to a realization
that this has just got to stop, I wasn't headed in the right direction
and something is obviously wrong with me. Of course I wasn't
there yet, it would still take some more medication and some
heavy self meditation, but thankfully I set myself on the path to
do this upon my release from jail.

I began attending outpatient therapy immediately, once
again. This was something I was compliant with 100% , once
again. I had not skipped a beat on my medicine either since I was
released from jail. I realized very quickly what had happened to
me and realize it had happened again. I was on the medication
"Abilify" during outpatient therapy, which seemed to be the one
drug that really made me snap out of my disillusioned reality. This
was the last pill that I ever took for anti psychotics, a miracle drug
for myself. While it may not work for everyone, I am sure glad it
did for me. I pondered constantly about what had happened to
me. While I felt embarrassed about my position in life and the
past few years, I also felt I had to overcome this. I wasn't sure if it
was going to happen again, but I wanted to do everything I could
to prevent it from occurring. All of these memories remained
fresh of how I acted, what I thought, what I saw, what I believed.
I spent time just thinking about what I hallucinated, why I thought
what I thought, my actions. *My God, I was an idiot.* Actually, I

knew that I wasn't, I knew something happened to me that I couldn't control, nor could I foresee it to prevent it. I feel I had made a mess of it and it was time for me to straighten it out the best I could. While it may not have been my entire fault, I believe I did not take any precautions necessary and was overly reckless during my rebellious era. As I began to better myself I ended up experimenting with letting off on the medication, slowly. I warned those that I loved to watch for signs, in case I ever started to drift back into that horrid state I came from. One thing I learned from this, at some point, I could not trust myself from what was actually true, if things were getting a little weird. During my therapy, I meditated a lot about my life and about life in general. I realized that at times I was a God. It was really fun to perceive myself as a divine being. I thought I'd never die, now I knew I had to face my inevitable mortality. Everything I experienced was rooted somewhere within me, my deepest darkest subconscious desires. I realized my personality traits of what I was played out in my actions. My child like state of innocence even came out at times, from years long gone. This was a pivotal moment in my life and I couldn't let my life continue going on this path, this path that made my life garbage. I came to a satisfactory conclusion of what is real for me. The universe and everything in society was now being understood in a new light, far from the former frame of reference that my Catholic indoctrination brought me. I rejected all that was belief based and began my path to where I am today. Today I realize I don't know a lot. I may not even know if my senses are failing me, but that's ok. A lot of people tend to have a lot of beliefs about things, but I like to stand on the fence a lot of the time. It's ok to know that I don't know and I don't need to believe in something just so I can close the door on that area. This is a complete 180 from where I was, when everything I wanted to be true was true.

Where any power of suggestion, the slightest hint, would become a hardcore fact that I would not only believe as real, but act off of, and dangerously so.

As mentioned previously, I ended up getting married to the woman who stood by my side through it all, Megan. It was quite the ride we both went through and if she stuck with me through all of that, I knew she was a keeper. I brushed up my resume and ended up getting a job that had an opportunity to become a career. I worked steadily at the new job and soon learned I was going to be a Dad. Now we have a beautiful daughter and I am a proud father and husband as well as a hard worker. I progressed in my job to become an Office Manager and have a key role in the organization that I work for. Nobody would ever think twice about my past and would be completely surprised to know what I have experienced in my early 20's.

Epilogue

Today, I still experience minor residual affects, mostly auditory hallucinations. Sometimes it is hard to know if what I am hearing is true. This only occurs when I hear background noise, such as loud crowds. I know it is the illness playing tricks on me when I hear people I don't know say something about me, yet they are out of normal listening range. Clues such as that help me understand what is occurring. This is something that nobody would know about me, as it doesn't affect me anymore on the same level it used to. I control it and it doesn't take me away on a long string of psychotic thoughts, because I am aware it is not real. Perhaps this can help those that experience these symptoms, although I understand everyone is different. If you experience similar symptoms as mine, I recommend being vigilant about everything you see and hear and question everything to verify if it is real. Be honest and open to your therapist as well as your family. Although I have not been on medication for the past 7 years, I do not recommend this for people who are suffering from these symptoms. I understand my situation is likely very unique in that the symptoms have diminished and are usually non existent. I hope if you suffer of mental illness that you too can find your path to a life based on reality and not delusions. I wonder how many religious miracles may be attributed solely to schizophrenic thoughts. Today I leave this story victorious, as I am accepted in society just as I was accepted in jail, but this time it is for all the right reasons.   Maybe there is something to Neitzsche's quote after all. My battle with monsters, the monsters inside me, was a lose/lose situation. This massive trial of life that I endured provided me with wisdom and oh so many lessons learned. Today I am almost grateful to have had the experience, although I know it held me back greatly. It affected me during college, a critical moment to the beginning of the rest of my life. My entire career and education was delayed. My state of mind afterwards, forever changed. For those who can identify with my experience, I hope you too can break free from the chains of your delusional reality.

For those who are struggling with mental illness of this nature, please take heed to these words of wisdom gained only through my own experience. Someone in a manic state of mine is suspect to turn and do the unexpected at any given moment. The less stimulation that is given to the manic individual, the better. Any sort of interaction from a simple "I love you" to the playing of music can trigger delusional thought. Someone in this state of mind is highly volatile and very dangerous. The best way to handle this is to get intervention immediately. The police will help, if you have to. Forceful intervention is sometimes needed. I can only thank medication for my recuperation today, however even though I have been off medicine for nearly 7 years at the time of publishing this book, I cannot say confidently that this will be the case with anybody. Each individual will handle mental illness differently and each mental illness is different in everyone's mind, regardless of similarities. For those of you who are struggling currently, my only advice is to please focus on finding the truth. The truth is all you need to set you free. While it may not agree, please take your medicine as well.

ABOUT THE AUTHOR

Mr. Markowski currently resides in Romeoville, Illinois, with his wife Megan and daughter Amelia. He works as a Manager at a packaging facility full time. Hobbies include playing with his daughter, traveling, playing basketball, playing guitar, preferring typical non psychotic activities.

For My Mother, her Eulogy.

Wings for Mom

I am not sure if I am able to do this, but I'm going to try, after all, Mom always said you don't know unless you try. This little light of mine, the strength that allows me to stand here now, that allows me to write and express this, is a gift Mom passed on to me, and I'm going to let it shine, to guide her safely and happily on her way home. This light of hers has been passed on to many, on to all of her children, we all have a little bit of her light, in all our unique ways and I know we're going to make sure that light is wrapped in love and given to our children, and the children of our children. That's going to be a lot of children.

While we are all saddened by Mom's passing, the great thing is that today we can celebrate her life, which was really very interesting. She shined brightly through the end of it all being constantly selfless and always still wanting the best for her children, grandchildren and her large, loving family. She truly had a light within that shone even in the face of imminent death. Our final conversation was one not so much about her, she just had to turn it around and make it about me, making sure that I lived the best life she saw for me. She was selfless and caring, motherly, and a fighter to the end.

I read a journal entry that Mom said her life was boring at some point, and she was ok with that. I believe she thought that only because she had a big imagination, a big powerful mind, that was capable of reaching for much more, and reach she did. While she may have been bored at points, she was most certainly not boring. When I told mom I was bored, she had quite the list for me to do. Read a book, stand on my head, draw, and clean your room. Mom did something about her own boredom too. She was highly opinionated, multi faceted, multi talented, a defender of the true and righteous, a headstrong warrior against injustice, all backed by her love of Jesus and unconditional love of everyone. She was a forgiver and an angel. She loved St. Michael the archangel, and I feel she and him have a lot in common. Mom was disgusted often, which she said regularly, not only during her last few months of being tired and having difficulty getting around, but really throughout all the time I knew her. She was disgusted by her perception of injustices and immorality of the world. We may or may not agree with what she stood for, I think we can all agree she fought for what she saw was good and holy and fought against all she saw as evil and immoral. A few of Mom's folders in her email show some of her concerned subjects. Religion, terrorists, politics, horses, down syndrome. I find it so funny that a 74 year old Grandmother would have a folder for her emails that just was in regard to terrorist activity. Yes, she was unique and watchful, passionate about so many things as well. Mom wanted a better life for all of us, not just her children, and that is what she fought for, for morality, for Jesus, for the betterment of mankind. She made her dent against her enemies and made me a proud son, for one. Even though I didn't always agree with her, I could openly discuss things with her. I loved our conversations on politics and the world, nature, life, and everything. She was a proud member of Eagle Forum, Birthright, the Hammond town council, and quite a bit of other organizations and causes. She really took a lot. She was after all, disgusted, fed up. It was all sickening. I understand this in her, she had such great empathy she could feel the pain she perceived in the world. Her medicine for that pain was her own beautiful mind and her drive to fix them.

How she affected us all, in her own little way, or in sometimes her big way, was not through her voice, which was somewhat quiet and some might say, even little, but through her actions and intent and meaning of words, her justice and fairness, unconditional love and the eyes to see what was right in the face of all that was wrong. The way she extinguished all her pain and anguishes that she has endured, to come out a fighter.

Not only that, Mom nurtured my intelligence, my sense of awe and wonder, my curiosity, my love of storms, science, everything and anything. She was a great writer, with beautiful elegant cursive, which was a reflection of who she was. Studious, self taught, she used to read every night. She read a lot, about politics and faith, her causes, stories of courage and honor. She subscribed to Readers Digest, read Ann Coulter and called in to political talk radio shows quite a bit, so much that she had some contacts of radio show hosts in her rolodex. She wrote so many letters to the editor, she ended up getting her own column a couple times in the Hammond Times, which you can see in her scrap book she left behind.

Mom was organized, she had so many things saved sometimes I think it might be because she knew she was forgetting things a lot. When you are interested in so many things it's easy to forget, but she was smart enough to take precautions to remember. I love this in her, who she was, because she was a good person with good intentions, very capable and easy to underestimate, because she was humble, smart, and cautious, but not too cautious. She was somewhat introverted and I know I got that from her as well. I understand her to be always thinking and making sure things were "good", as in moral.

Mom was a great drawer and that never died in her. She was great at drawing faces, people, and horses, something that many find to be the most difficult, including me. I saw some of her drawings from this past year, and they looked like they did from over 30 years ago. I imagine her drawing, all alone one night, at her old age... If only I could've been outside looking in, watching her draw, seeing a sweet little smile come across her face when she knew she still had it, because knowing mom, she did just that.

Not only did she do all this, she raised or helped raise 6 children and treated the Markowski children as her own as well, caring for Janice in all the time she could, her loving unselfish way is something to challenge us all. Mom passed down to us so many good things, just in actions alone. And those things came back around, especially in her last few years. Her life was redeemed and made pleasant, exciting and comfortable by my lovely sisters, who took great effort to care for her in her dire time of need.

Every time I look up in the sky and see the stars, I think of Mom. She always looked at the stars, those stars up there are very special for her and me. And it's something so little, to say, "look at the stars, they're beautiful tonight"... but it became something so much more, forever more. The light of those stars for me represent her awe and wonder, her beautiful curiosity. I always have her in my mind when I look up at the starry night sky. That light of hers, penetrating through so those injustices almost as numerous as the stars themselves, was tested in fire for long enough, give her her wings, she earned them.

For my Father, his Eulogy.

On the night my father died I was walking mom up the stairs and waiting for her to unlock the door, I saw a fox running down 167th street right in front of our house. I have never seen a fox in Hessville, Hammond, or any other street in America for that matter. Of course dad used to hunt all sorts of animals, including fox. That night driving home it was a little comforting remembering seeing that fox run down our street that night. Perhaps it was the animal world paying homage to an old worthy foe, or maybe even something more, or perhaps nothing significant at all, but it may be significant to some, so I thought I would share this morning.

Dad loved talking about his glory days of hunting when he was younger, hunting all day all over Northwest Indiana, running through the vast fields and forests, some of which are now long gone and replaced by shopping centers or subdivisions. He would come home to the farm for home cooked meals. Running in those fields all day got him very hungry, and he would work up an appetite. And, yes he could run too – he could "run like the wind" he would say. I'm sure he could, from working on a farm all day and hunting animals down, he must have been a great athlete as well as a great hunter, and I loved waking up early in the morning to go hunting, I could feel the excitement and I knew my dad knew what he was doing. He taught me that you could also hunt mushrooms. Hunt mushrooms? Apparently, you need to know what you're doing, where to find them, which ones to get. He'd come home with buckets and buckets of mushrooms. I didn't like them back then, but they did smell good. He was a great outdoorsman. He knew how to work the land. He had a nice small garden which I have the fond memory of getting vegetables and bringing them for mom to cook for dinner. He also had the greenest lawn in the area. He was outside watering his lawn every night in the summer, just standing there with the hose. I never knew why then, but I know now that he took pride in his lawn. It was work after all, and there is honor in work, even something as simple as taking care of your lawn. He knew and taught me that it increases the land value, not only for us, but for the whole neighborhood. He was a dedicated, hard working man, and he worked as long as he could physically do so.

As long as I can remember, I always beat him in arm wrestling. But, I know he let me win when I was younger. That's what dad's do. I always loved wrestling with my dad. Even when he was too old and arthritis was tearing through his bones, he still gave it a shot but it was too easy then. But I kept on him, even at the nursing home in his final months I tried riling him up for an old arm wrestling match, just for laughs and old time's sake. I think I got a little smile out of him. He loved playing Checkers, electronic battleship, and ping pong. I don't think he ever refused a challenge from me. Not even at the nursing home, when he could barely move the pieces on his own, he gave it a try. At one point he was beating me there, here he is barely able to talk and he had one more piece than me, and I was good at checkers! But he taught me everything I knew. We played hundreds upon hundreds of checkers games. I wasn't taking it easy on him either, but we couldn't finish because it was a bit too much for him, and I knew. I was just glad to be able to squeeze a few more moves in with him.

I don't know how many times people thought dad was my grandfather, but I never had any problem of correcting them as long as I could remember. After all we were "buddies" and we'd go everywhere together. We often went out to eat, at Chuck and Irene's for fish dinners on Fridays, or Ponderosa or Sizzler on the weekends. Some other old favorites were Pepe's and House of Pizza. He'd take us shopping to Southlake Mall, Woodmar Mall and anywhere in between.

He always bought the top of the line stuff, he taught me that too because the stuff that was cheap often broke and ended up being more expensive in the long run. He taught me a lot of things, some things I still haven't quite yet grasped, after all he has a good 50 years on me and I'm on my first, but somehow he always provided for his very large family. I think when he was my age he was running a house with, what, 6 kids already? I'm not sure exactly, but I know I couldn't hold a candle up to him in that department. This man grew up during the end of the Great Depression; he must've learned a trick or too going through that. I couldn't really imagine what that was like. At the time of writing this I am on my computer at home with my duo 2.0 GHZ computer processors with a 23" widescreen computer monitor. Yet my dad had to help his dad sell newspapers in Chicago so they had food on the table. I know my dad didn't have it as easy as I did and I know that I wouldn't want to walk in his shoes, I know he dad was loving in that he wanted me to live a better life than he did, as all good dads would want.

Growing up, we always had food on the table. He was a great cook alongside Mom. He could make some great dishes and some not so great dishes also. Some of us might remember his Spanish Pork Chops, or the Tripe soup, or Czarnina (duck blood soup). When my friends asked what we were having for supper and my dad said Walleye, they laughed as if we were "weird". After all, what little kid in Hessville eats Walleye for dinner? Well I guess if you're parents were 40-50 years older than you, you did. That was some of the benefits of having old fashioned parents, they didn't have frozen foods growing up, they had to cook real meals. But, then again, I was always skinny. From looking at those old pictures of him when he was around my age, I think I definitely got some of that from him.

Many of us remember the many camping trips we went on. My dad took us camping so much I can't remember everywhere we went. There are many memories from camping, fishing on Lake Michigan. I had the greatest Lake perch in my life from fish we caught off the lake in Cedar Falls Michigan. Dad knew how to gut them, something I never got the guts to do myself, and we'd cook them on the grill. He could do stuff like that, something I learned to admire. He did a lot of thing I was always a little squeamish about. Like tearing the skins off of squirrels we hunt and then eating them. I grew up in a different era, and some of my peers wouldn't ever imagine eating squirrel, but you definitely learn a few tricks living with someone who passes for your Grandfather.

Dad took me all over the nation, I can't remember every place we've been to, but the ones that stick out are Raccoon Lake, Turkey Run, Cooperstown, the air force museum, Washington DC, and the California trip... which I'm told I was too young to remember, but I think I might have a few vague memories, like the old Station wagon overheating out there in the middle of the hot sun, and some freezing nights in the pop up in some unknown state out West. He showed me as much of the world as he could through traveling and I always appreciated it.

How he had the money to do it, I'll never really know. I'll never know how he supported so many children. He found a way - Just like I must now. Whenever I feel like not going to work at 5:30 in the morning let me just think of my dad working all sorts of odd hours in the mill for 38 years straight. I don't think that was an easy job either, being a millwright. But he must've been good at it. He was always fixing something around the house. He had so many tools that it would take me a lifetime to even get to know what they all did, let alone know how to use them. Many times I remember going to Lindys hardware to pick up something, because something was always broke. I think he could nearly fix anything, until he got older when his hands failed him. When that happens, he and the dad from "A Christmas Story" seem all too similar, however some of the curse words he came up with, were, well... you know. And he had a voice on him; it was possibly the loudest voice I've ever heard in my life. He could scream at me from at least 4 blocks away and I would hear him and I knew he knew I heard him too, no matter how often I attempted to ignore it. When you get yelled at that loud, you have no choice but to come home.

Throughout my life, I learned that I should've listened to my dad more. I guess we all do this and end up going our own way, then coming back. The prodigal son isn't famous for nothing. But there are many things this old man has taught and will teach me. There's still a lot to learn, he left me with so many stories that they will resonate as long as I can remember, partly because he told me every story dozens if not hundreds of times.

I realized after growing up that dad had his own way of doing things which was much different than the rest of the worlds. There are many lessons I have learned and will still continue to learn from my dad. I know if I look hard enough, there are lessons about sacrifice in my dad. Lessons about honor, courage and strength. This is what a father is for and while we had our hard times, we wouldn't know the good times from the bad if the hard times weren't there. There are many things I appreciate in my dad; he was unique in every way I could imagine. He left his imprints on me in many ways and if there's any good qualities that may come from me at any given time, yes mom you could be most definitely be the reason, but some things only a father can teach a son, and with the passing of dad perhaps I hope all of you could continue to see the good qualities of my father here and there in me, if I'm capable of learning and executing them. And hopefully, I'll be able to pass something on that may be a different for this day and age, just like dad did. He always gave everyone something to think about.

www.ingramcontent.com/pod-product-compliance
Lightning Source LLC
Chambersburg PA
CBHW030909180526
45163CB00004B/1763